Niveditha S. Prasad
M. Sheejith
Raj V. S. Sarath
and Nivea T. Francis

Digital Implant Planning and Guided Implant Surgery

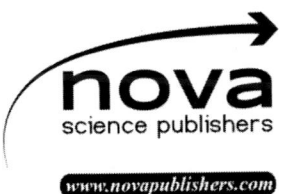

Copyright © 2024 by Nova Science Publishers, Inc.

https://doi.org/10.52305/GDQO4706

All rights reserved. No part of this book may be reproduced, stored in a retrieval system or transmitted in any form or by any means: electronic, electrostatic, magnetic, tape, mechanical photocopying, recording or otherwise without the written permission of the Publisher.

We have partnered with Copyright Clearance Center to make it easy for you to obtain permissions to reuse content from this publication. Please visit copyright.com and search by Title, ISBN, or ISSN.

For further questions about using the service on copyright.com, please contact:

	Copyright Clearance Center	
Phone: +1-(978) 750-8400	Fax: +1-(978) 750-4470	E-mail: info@copyright.com

NOTICE TO THE READER

The Publisher has taken reasonable care in the preparation of this book but makes no expressed or implied warranty of any kind and assumes no responsibility for any errors or omissions. No liability is assumed for incidental or consequential damages in connection with or arising out of information contained in this book. The Publisher shall not be liable for any special, consequential, or exemplary damages resulting, in whole or in part, from the readers' use of, or reliance upon, this material. Any parts of this book based on government reports are so indicated and copyright is claimed for those parts to the extent applicable to compilations of such works.

Independent verification should be sought for any data, advice or recommendations contained in this book. In addition, no responsibility is assumed by the Publisher for any injury and/or damage to persons or property arising from any methods, products, instructions, ideas or otherwise contained in this publication.

This publication is designed to provide accurate and authoritative information with regards to the subject matter covered herein. It is sold with the clear understanding that the Publisher is not engaged in rendering legal or any other professional services. If legal or any other expert assistance is required, the services of a competent person should be sought. FROM A DECLARATION OF PARTICIPANTS JOINTLY ADOPTED BY A COMMITTEE OF THE AMERICAN BAR ASSOCIATION AND A COMMITTEE OF PUBLISHERS.

Library of Congress Cataloging-in-Publication Data

ISBN: 979-8-89113-324-2

Published by Nova Science Publishers, Inc. † New York

Contents

Foreword vii
 M. Ranjith

Acknowledgments ix

Chapter 1 **Introduction** 1

Chapter 2 **History** 7
 Historical Overview in Brief 9

Chapter 3 **Evolution of Guided Implant Surgery** 11

Chapter 4 **Goals of Guided Implant Surgery** 17

Chapter 5 **Indications of Guided Implant Surgery** 19
 Planning for Three or More Implants in a Row 19
 Proximity to Important Anatomic Structures 20
 Problems Related to the Proximity
 of Adjacent Teeth 20
 Questionable Bone Volume 21
 Implant Position: Critical to the Restoration 21

Chapter 6 **Advantages of Guided Implant Surgery** 23

Chapter 7 **Disadvantages of Guided Implant Surgery** 27

Chapter 8 **Guided Implant Surgery Systems** 29

Chapter 9 **Guided Surgical Templates** 35

Chapter 10 **Types of Surgical Templates** 43
 Universal Master Sleeves 44
 Manufacturer-Specific Master Sleeves 45
 Universal Templates (Pilot Surgiguide,
 Universal Surgiguide) 46
 Manufacturer-Specific Guide (SAFE SurgiGuide) 47

Contents

Customized Conventional Radiographic
Surgical Template:...48
    Fabrication Process 48
Computer-Generated Surgical Template 50
    Procedures for the Fabrication
    of Stereolithographic Templates..................... 50
Double Scan Protocol 52
Making a Computer-Aided Template 52

Chapter 11   **Surgical Application of Templates** 55
Nonlimiting Design 57
Completely Limiting Design 57

Chapter 12   **Advantages and Disadvantages of Templates** 59

Chapter 13   **Protocols for Guided Implant Surgery** 61
Access to a Cone-Beam CT Scanner...............................61
Implant Planning Software 61
A Surgical Template...62
Guided Implant Surgery Drill Kit...................................62

Chapter 14   **Guided Implant Surgery**..63
Surgical Procedure in Brief 65
Guided Implant Placement 68

Chapter 15   **CT Based Guided Implant Surgery** 69
Data Acquisitions 69
Identification..69
Registration..70
Navigation 70

Chapter 16   **CAD Cam Based Guided Implant Surgery** 71
Technique 71
Surgical Procedure...74

Chapter 17   **Cast Based Guided Implant Surgery** 77

Chapter 18   **CBCT Guided Flapless Implant Surgery** 83
Surgical Procedures 84
    Pre-Operative Instructions............................... 84
    Free-Handed Surgery.. 84
    Pilot-Drill-Guided Surgery 85
    Fully-Guided Surgery....................................... 85
    Post-Operative Instructions.............................. 86

Contents

	Post-Operative CBCT	86
	Prosthetic Procedures	86
Chapter 19	**Image Guided Implant Surgery**	87
	Surgical Accuracy	90
	Fabrication and Guide Seating	91
	In-Office Guide Printing	92
	Complications	92
	Robotic Surgery	93
	When to Use Image-Guided Surgery	93
Chapter 20	**Printed Surgical Template for Guided Implant Surgery**	95
	Virtual Template Design	95
Chapter 21	**One Abutment One Time**	99
	Treatment Plan	99
	Surgical Procedure	101
	Postoperative Treatment	102
Chapter 22	**Teeth in an Hour**	105
Chapter 23	**Clinical Outcome of Guided Implant Surgery**	107
	Implant Survival	107
	Accuracy	108
	Complications	109
Chapter 24	**Artificial Intelligence and Guided Implant Surgery**	111
Chapter 25	**Conclusion**	115
About the Authors		117
Index		121

Foreword

M. Ranjith
Prof., Dr., KUHS University, Kerala, India

As digital technology is conquering our day to day activities guided implant surgery will be the future of implant dentistry and will not become outdated in this digital world so fast. Conventional free hand implant surgery has been performed by dental implant surgeons since the introduction of osseointergrated dental implants and there are many books which give information regarding conventional free hand implant surgery. But this book which deals with guided implant surgery involves a reverse engineering workflow, which establishes the ideal position and morphology of the planned restoration and then virtually plan the ideal position of dental implant according to the planned restoration.

For the beginners this book offers the way to mastering the hands on skills of digital dentistry. The practioners will find useful its information on advanced digital implant planning. Both will also gain insight into the theory behind digital implant planning and guided implant surgery.

The authors have researched many aspects of digital implant planning and have written widely on the subject.

Acknowledgments

We would like to acknowledge the publisher, editors, friends and support staff at Kmct Dental College. They were very helpful in the various stages of developing and publishing this book. We would also like to express our sincere gratitude to all our family members.

Chapter 1

Introduction

The field of implant prosthodontics has made significant advancements since the initial presentation of Brånemark's osseointegration concepts to the dental profession in the early 1980s. We have witnessed a dramatic shift in all areas of this biotechnology's application, including the advancements in both the macro- and micro-design of implants, with over 300 implant manufacturers currently offering various products. Exciting changes have also occurred in materials science and using CAD/CAM manufacturing for titanium and zirconia abutments, along with one-piece, fixed partial-denture substructures. Further, we have evolved from the original two-stage surgical protocols, as described by Brånemark, to the concepts of immediate placement and immediate loading (where indicated). We have seen the development of both soft and hard tissue grafting techniques and technologies, such as guided bone regeneration techniques (GBR), that use different resorbable and non-resorbable membrane technologies and a variety of allografts and xenografts. We have seen block grafts, sinus grafts, distraction osteogenesis, platelet-enriched plasma (PRP), and the application of bone morphogenic proteins (BMP 2) with various carriers. Another notable advancement in this field has been guided surgery, which uses sophisticated three-dimensional implant planning software programs in conjunction with either fan beam (CT) or cone beam radiographic scanning technology [1].

In the past, there were many problems with the placement of endosseous implants, such as patient movement while drilling, limited surgery time due to the use of local anaesthesia, limited visibility of the operation field, mental transfer of two-dimensional radiographs into the three-dimensional surgical environment, and aesthetic, biomechanical, and functional limitations of the prosthetic treatment. Thus, with limited time and a restricted view, the surgeon must make numerous decisions while nurturing a conscious patient under aseptic conditions. Therefore, a thorough preoperative planning of the number of implants to be placed and their size, position, and inclination will free the surgeon's mind, allowing the surgeon to focus on the patient and tissue management [2].

With the recent introduction of new three-dimensional (3D) diagnostic and treatment planning technologies in implant dentistry, a team-based approach to the planning and implantation of dental implants, based on a restoratively-driven treatment plan, has become the standard for providing quality patient care. The team can begin with the desired outcome, the planned tooth, and then place an implant in the precise location following the restoration plan. The precise and predictable placement of implants following a computer-generated virtual treatment plan is now a reality, bringing the virtual plan from the computer to the patient. Recent advances in 3D imaging in dentistry, in combination with the introduction of third-party proprietary implant planning software and associated surgical instrumentation, have revolutionized the diagnosis and treatment of dental implants and created an interdisciplinary environment where communication improves patient care and outcomes [3].

Implant-supported oral restorations have become an increasingly popular treatment option for partially edentulous and completely edentulous patients, as well as in patients with severe bone loss and in locations that were previously not considered for implant placement but have been made possible utilizing bone augmentation, regeneration, and soft tissue regeneration procedures [4]. Earlier implants were placed only in the area with a significant amount of bone, regardless of the placement of the final definitive restoration. The result was that the implant placement was not as accurate as intended. Even a minor variation caused difficulties in the fabrication of the final prostheses. It was discovered that failure occurred due to insufficient anatomical consideration during the pre-surgical phase. Accurate implant placement is required to achieve the best functional and aesthetic result. It can be effectively achieved through a surgical guide that provides adequate information regarding implant placement and, at the time of surgery, fits onto the existing dentition or the edentulous span [5].

Implant dentistry is entering its second half-century after gaining a solid foothold as a predictable means of tooth replacement. Today, the focus on osseointegration is diminishing, and the emphasis on nature-like tooth replacement, minimally invasive surgical and restorative techniques, and efficiencies of time and cost is increasing. A "crown-down" approach to treatment planning and implant positioning is necessary to achieve these goals because implant position can no longer solely depend on bone availability. With the end result in mind, the surgeon is expected to place the implant in the appropriate position, at a reasonable and safe depth, and with proper angulation to facilitate efficient, lifelike tooth replacement.

The risks associated with Malpositioned implants include functional and aesthetic problems. Buser et al. pointed out that a successful esthetic outcome can only be achieved with "an ideal implant position in all three dimensions." They described proper implant position as a zone within the buccolingual, mesiodistal, and apico-coronal dimensions rather than a specific point. By placing the implant within these "comfort zones," a functional and aesthetic outcome can be predicted. A violation of the comfort zone may result in complications such as peri-implant bone resorption followed by soft-tissue recession and esthetic failure. Pre-surgical, crown-down digital planning in conjunction with guided implant surgery is an ideal means to accurately and precisely position an implant within the comfort zone and avoid complications [6].

Guided implant surgery is a procedure in which precision surgical instrumentation is used with three-dimensional CT images [7]. Marquardt, Witkowski, and Strub concluded: "It is now possible to predetermine the precise three-dimensional position of the planned implant before the actual implant insertion and to transfer this position to the surgical site. This increases the quality of both the surgical procedure and the restoration" [8]. However, three-dimensional radiographic imaging for dental implant treatment planning can be a seemingly complex and daunting process [9]. Implant positions are based on pre-surgical diagnostic imaging, study models, and diagnostic wax-ups for the planned tooth replacement. The surgical guide between the diagnostic information and the patient is often an acrylic stent, which may or may not have precise guide channels for implant positioning [10].

Hämmerle et al. published the consensus on indications and clinical recommendations for CAD/CAM procedures in implant dentistry. In this consensus, they defined the term guided surgery, which consists of using a static guide that reproduces the virtual position of the implant to allow for intraoperative real-time tracking of the drills according to the planned trajectory [11]. Many of these techniques are already available in clinical practice and are on their way to becoming routine treatment options. It is of great importance to evaluate the accuracy, which is defined as the deviations in location or angle between the virtual planning of computer-guided surgery and dental implant placements [12].

Although digitally designing the ideal implant location, position, and angulation is essential, achieving it during surgical procedures is a prerequisite for treatment success. Traditionally, radiographic images have been used as the basis for handmade drill guides for implant placement. However, these guides often could not account for proper implant depth and were prone to the inconsistencies inherent in analogue fabrication methods. With the advent of CBCT imaging and treatment planning software, anatomical information can be incorporated into the implant placement and restorative plan, and more precise, CAM-fabricated surgical stents can be produced. Such patient-specific, computer-generated, and machined surgical stents allow dentists to place implants more accurately and efficiently, at the proper location and angulation, and to the proper depth. The implementation of digital technology in patient care has empowered us to deliver precise and personalized implant restorations with unprecedented speed [13].

The concept of guided implant surgery permits the surgeon, restorative dentist, and laboratory to collaborate on each implant patient's diagnosis and treatment planning. The three-dimensional computer model of the patient's oral structures allows all team members to evaluate various factors, including the available bone for implant placement, the proximity of the placement site to adjacent dentition, existing implants, the maxillary sinus, and the inferior alveolar nerve. This assessment can be conducted with ease [14]. The utilization of image-guided surgery initially emerged within the field of neurosurgery and has subsequently been extended to encompass a wide range of medical and dental interventions.

References

[1] Dunn DB. Guided implant surgery - The new "standard of care?" *Australasian Dental Practice.* January/February 2009.

[2] Vercruyssen M, Laleman I, Jacobs R, Quirynen M. Computer-supported implant planning and guided surgery: A narrative review. *Clin Oral Impl Res.* 2015;26 (Suppl. 11):69–76.

[3] Gary Orentlicher MA. Guided surgery for implant therapy. *Oral Maxillofacial Surg Clin N Am.* 2011; 23:239–256.

[4] Widmann G BR. Accuracy in computer-aided implant surgery: A review. *Int J Oral Maxillofac Implants.* 2006; 21:305-13.

[5] Rohit Shah. Guided implant surgery. *Int Educ Res J.* 2017;3(11).

[6] Norkin FJ. *Assessing image-guided implant surgery in today's clinical practice.* 2013.

[7] Richard H. Yamada DVG. Guided implant surgery. *"A Periodontal Practice Committed to Excellence."* 2013.

[8] Al Me. *Three-dimensional navigation surgery.* Dental council of North America.

[9] Scherer M. CAD/CAM guided surgery in implant dentistry. *Alpha Omega Int Dent Fraternity.* 2014.

[10] Navigation surgery. *Dental council of North America.*
[11] Giorgio Andrea Dolcini MCaC. Guided surgery to final prosthesis with a fully digital procedure: A prospective clinical study. *Int J Dent.* 2016.
[12] Tardieu PB. *The art of computer -guided implantology.* Quintessence Publishing.
[13] Mirzayan A. *CBCT and digital technology for prosthetically driven and guided implant placement surgery.* 2017.
[14] Pozzi A, Polizzi G, Moy PK. Guided surgery with tooth-supported templates for single missing teeth: A critical review. *Eur J Oral Implantol.* 2016;9 Suppl 1: S35-53.

Chapter 2

History

Since the invention of the first dental radiographs, dentists have acquired a sense of ease in assessing and diagnosing patients using two-dimensional (2D) pictures, such as periapical, bitewing, panoramic, and cephalometric radiographs. Because there were so few alternatives, clinicians had to accept the apparent limitations of these technologies in evaluating 3D problems. Because of their hospital-based training, oral and maxillofacial surgeons have long used computed tomography (CT) scans for the 3D evaluation of facial trauma and pathologic lesions. These CT evaluations were typically viewed in 2D as axial or reformatted frontal or coronal slices through the area of interest of a patient's anatomy, printed on plain films, or viewed as such on a computer screen. The rest of the dentistry community had little to no experience with 3D picture evaluation [1].

In 1987, computed tomography (CT) was introduced into dentistry to add another dimension to dental implant treatment planning. This technology allowed clinicians, for the first time, to evaluate anatomic structures with a higher level of accuracy. In 1999, dental implant planning applications were developed, allowing interactive planning of virtual implants in 2-D and 3-D. The first medical-grade helical CT scanners were exclusively single-slice equipment with slower operational speeds. These devices were mainly situated within hospitals or privately-owned radiology clinics. Today's typical medical multi-slice CT scanners can scan the upper and/or lower jaw in a few seconds. However, their size and cost, radiation exposure, lack of familiarity and training among dentists, and perceived cost/benefit ratio in patient care make them unsuitable for use in a dental office setting. Cone beam volumetric tomography (CBVT) or cone beam computed tomography (CBCT) was first presented to the dental community in 1998 with the creation and release of the New Tom 9000 (Quantitative Radiology, Verona, Italy). Although the first machines were larger than those available today, the advantages were that they produced good 3D images at lower radiation doses, and the footprint of the machines was small enough to fit into a dental office. The disadvantages were that, although the radiation was less than medical-grade CT, it was more than conventional dental radiographs. Because of the reduced radiation, the images produced had less definition than medical CT. Since the debut of the first CBCT, numerous manufacturers have created and released machines with various unique features. The gold standard for accurate 3D diagnosis continues to be medical-grade CT. The recent introduction of adaptive statistical iterative reconstruction (ASIR) software has been reported to allow up to a 50% radiation dose reduction in medical CT scans without diminishing image quality. Each CBCT scanner has a unique average deviation and percentage error measurement [2].

Computed tomography (CT) was the subsequent advancement, along with relatively simple planning software such as Dentascan, which utilized a variety of simple radiographic templates. At this stage of the development of implant prosthodontics, it must be considered that most of the cases were fully edentulous (and mainly in the mandible), and the emphasis at that time was on function rather than aesthetics. Indeed, early on, there was very little sophistication in abutment options, and single and partial cases were rarely attempted. In the late 1980s, articles began to appear in the literature discussing the use of DentaScans to evaluate the bone of the maxilla and mandible in preparation for the placement of dental implants. Columbia Scientific (CSI) introduced 3D Dental software in 1988. This software converted CT axial slices into reformatted cross-sectional images of the alveolar ridges for diagnosis and evaluation. In 1991, a combination software was introduced, ImageMaster-101, which allowed the additional feature of placing graphic dental implants on the cross-sectional images. The first version of Sim/Plant was introduced by CSI in 1993, allowing the placement of virtual implants of exact dimensions on CT images in cross-sectional, axial, and panoramic views. In 1999, Simplant 6.0 was introduced, adding the creation of 3D reformatted image surface rendering to the software [1].

In 2000, Professor Jacobs of the Oral Imaging Cluster at KU Leuven compared the accuracy of implant placement using simple drill guides, manual placement without a guide or template, and meticulous care utilizing cadavers. The accuracy level in the X-axis obtained with implants placed utilizing drill guides was 0.92 mm, as opposed to manual placement with an error of 3.71 mm. It is important to note that these implants were placed under "ideal conditions," with no saliva, blood, tongue, opening issues, etc. In 2002, Professor Daniel van Steenberghe published a paper titled "A custom template and definitive prosthesis allowing immediate implant loading in the Maxilla: a clinical report" in the *International Journal of Oral and Maxillofacial Implants*. He presented data on two cadavers and eight human subjects utilizing LITORIM—Leuven Information Technology-based Oral

Rehabilitation using Implants. Here he compared the results of the implant positions and axes achieved from the positions planned versus those achieved, following the use of computer tomography scanning technology and a sophisticated three-dimensional software planning program and surgical templates produced from this planning process. This technology formed the basis of what we now know as NobelGuide. He concluded that "the results indicated nearly a perfect match between the positions and axes of the placed implants and those planned." The error in the implant axes was $1.8°$ with a standard deviation of 1, while the error in the implant entry point was 0.8 mm with a standard deviation of 0.3. These results were very encouraging for precision implant prosthodontics [3]. A completely redesigned upgrade of the NobelGuide software, NobelClinician, was introduced in 2011. Software from other manufacturers, such as EasyGuide (Keystone Dental, Burlington, MA, USA), Straumann coDiagnostiX (Straumann, Basel, Switzerland), VIP Software (BioHorizons, Birmingham, AL, USA), Implant Master (IDent, Foster City, CA, USA), and others, is now available as well. Other implant manufacturers have developed instrument trays for the guided placement of their implants using the Simplant software for implant planning (i.e., Facilitate, AstraTech Dental, Molndal, Sweden; Navigator, Biomet 3i, Palm Beach Gardens, FL, USA; ExpertEase, Dentsply Friadent, Mannheim, Germany) [1].

Historical Overview in Brief

- In late 1980 - DentScans
- In 1988 - Columbia Scientific (CSI) introduced 3D Dental
- In 1991 - a combination software ImageMaster 101
- In 1993 - the first version of Simplant was introduced by CSI.
- In 1999 - Simplant 6.0 was introduced.
- In 2001 - Materialise (Leuven, Belgium) purchased CSI.
- In 2002 - introduced the technology of drilling osteotomies to exact depth and direction through a surgical guide.
- In 2005 - NobelBiocare (Zurich, Switzerland) introduced NobelProcera/NobelGuide.
- In 2011 - a completely redesigned upgrade of NobelGuide software, NobelClinician was introduced
- Now the softwares also available are

- Easy guide (Keystone Dental,USA)
- Straumann coDiagnostiX(Straumann,Switzerland)
- VIP Software (Biohorizons,USA)
- Implant Master (Ident, USA)
- Other manufacturers have developed instrument trays for guided placement of their implants using Simplant software.
  - Facilitate (AstraTech Dental,Sweden)
  - Navigator (Biomet 3i, USA)
  - ExpertEase(Dentsply Friadent,Germany)

References

[1] Pozzi A, Polizzi G, Moy PK. Guided surgery with tooth-supported templates for single missing teeth: A critical review. *Eur J Oral Implantol*. 2016;9 Suppl 1: S35-53.

[2] Nejat R. Computer-guided dental implant surgery: Evolving, efficient, esthetic. *J dentistry*. 2011.

[3] Dunn DB. Guided implant surgery - The new "standard of care?" *Australasian Dental Practice*. January/February 2009.

Chapter 3

Evolution of Guided Implant Surgery

Since the first dental implant surgery by Brånemark in the early 1960s, the evolution of surgical techniques and the fine-tuning of surgical methodology have allowed for more predictable results with desirable esthetic outcomes. With the advent of guided implant surgery, implant placement and restoration success rates have continued to improve. Examination of the implant site and reflection upon the evolution of guided surgery for the completely edentulous arch allows for continued improvement in implant placement and prosthesis success for patients and practitioners. The utilization of computer-generated surgical guides has demonstrated potential advantages in enhancing the precision of implant placement. However, it is crucial to acknowledge that the accuracy of surgical guides depends on the accuracy with which the virtual planning is transferred to the actual surgical site. An understanding of how virtual implant planning software transfers the positions of the planned implant sites to a computer-aided design or computer-aided manufacturing (CAD/CAM) surgical guide is essential. Position transfer occurs in two ways: one is "surface mapping." Surface mapping is based on a cast of the patient and computed tomography (CT) data. Using the gathered information, the program matches numerous points on the surface of the cast to the corresponding anatomical surface points in the CT data. Proper mapping between the image data and the physical space allows for producing an accurate CAD/CAM surgical guide. In order to avoid inaccuracies in surface mapping registration, accurate impressions and casts must be made to create a precise mechanical fit of the templates in the patient's mouth. The second technique for position transfer uses fiduciary or radiopaque markers in a radiographic template for dual scanning. Two CT scans are subsequently taken: the first is of the patient wearing the radiographic template, and the second is of the radiographic template only. Based on the automated matching positions of the fiducial markers, the two scans are superimposed. The surgical template can then be fabricated using the scanned radiographic template as a reference. A key advantage of using a radiographic template is seeing the planned implant position and restorative tooth positions in an overlay of the patient's CT data or anatomy.

Whenever new technologies are implemented into traditional practice, it is crucial to determine the extent to which the technology is of benefit. In vitro and in vivo studies should be examined to evaluate the new techniques and technologies. In studies comparing the accuracy of implant implantation using stereolithographic surgical guides on epoxy mandibles, CAD/CAM templates were compared to conventionally fabricated templates. Comparisons between the virtual plans for implant placement and the actual placement of implants showed a greater than average deviation in surgical placement using a traditional template compared to a CAD/CAM template. The distance between the centre of the head of the planned and actual implant varied by 1.5 ± 0.7 mm for the traditional template and 0.9 ± 0.5 mm for the CAD/CAM template. The distance between the centre of the apex of the planned and actual implants varied by 2.1 ± 0.97 mm for the traditional template and by 1.0 ± 0.6 mm for the CAD/CAM template. The angle formed between the long axis of the planned and actual implant varied by 8.0 ± 4.5 degrees for the traditional template and by 4.5 ± 2.0 degrees for the CAD/CAM template. Based on the present studies, research suggests that CAD/CAM templates increase accuracy.

Furthermore, studies show that CAD/CAM surgical templates allow for the ideal placement of multiple implants and enable the modification of prosthetically driven implant positioning based on anatomic limitations. Although studies show a higher accuracy for CAD/CAM surgical templates over traditional ones, exploring studies comparing planned implant placement to actual implant placement using soft tissue-borne CAD/CAM surgical templates is essential. The accuracy of NobelGuide surgical templates (manufactured by Nobel Biocare, Zurich) was investigated in a study that involved comparing the actual placement of 10 implants in the fully edentulous maxilla of two cadaver jaws with their planned placement. By employing fiducially linked markers, a comparative analysis was conducted on presurgical and postsurgical CT images, which unveiled significant proximity between the intended placement and the observed site of the implants. On average, there was 0.8 mm of deviation between the planned and placed implant at the head of the implant, 0.9 mm of deviation at the apex of the implant, and a 1.8-degree deviation of implant placement relative to the angle at which the implant was planned to be placed. In addition to increasing the accuracy of implant position placement, studies show that using CT scans and surgical planning software yields a high implant survival rate. When surgical planning software and CT scans were used to create a fixed prosthesis for an immediate load treatment, there was a 92 per cent survival rate of implants over a period of 24 months. Although the potential with CAD/CAM templates for precise implant placement exists, there is still variation in the degree of accuracy with computer-generated templates. Very few clinical studies use CAD/CAM—surgical templates to evaluate implant placement accuracy. In one study, CAD/CAM was used to fabricate multiple bone and tooth-borne templates for different twist drills of sizes 2.2 mm, 3.2 mm, and 4.0 mm. SimPlant (DENTSPLY Implants, Waltham, Mass.) was applied according to the SurgiGuide protocol. Based on preoperative and postoperative CT scans, the deviation at the head of the implant was 2.45 ± 1.42 mm with a range of 0.2–4.5 mm, the deviation at the apex of the implant was 2.99 ± 1.77 mm with a range of 0.8–7.1 mm, and the angular comparison was 7.25 ± 2.67 degrees with a range of 3.6–12.2 degrees. Additional studies continue to show variations in the accuracy of implant placement.

A clinical study using computed tomography-based NobelGuide surgical templates and NobelGuide protocols looked at the variation in the accuracy of implant placement. To assess implant placement accuracy, patients had post-insertion scans using a triple-scan technique: template scan, template and patient preplacement scan, and template and patient postplacement scan. Measurements were made with the fused implants using Adobe Photoshop. X- and Z-axis average values were obtained at the shoulder and apex of the implant. Planning varied from placement in the shoulder X-axis by 0.46 mm (maximum 1.42 mm), in the shoulder Y-axis by 0.43 mm (maximum 1.5 mm), and in the shoulder Z-axis by 0.53 mm (maximum 1.85 mm). Regarding the apices, on the X-axis, there was a difference of 0.7 mm (maximum 1.84 mm). On the Y-axis, a difference of 0.59 mm (maximum 1.89 mm), and on the Z-axis, a difference of 0.52 mm (maximum 2.02 mm). The angular deviation was 3.53 degrees (maximum 8.1 degrees). With the understanding that variation in the accuracy of implant placement using computer-generated surgical guides exists, it is important to examine data using a reliable system that can give a practitioner insight into how the accuracy of CAD/CAM surgical templates can be maximized. The first NobelGuide treatments in North America were reported in the *Journal of the California Dental Association* in 2003 and have been tracked to validate and learn from the procedure. Since the first cases, multiple patients have been treated, and their cases have been recorded. In addition to the pioneer studies, in vivo and in vitro studies provide helpful information for the practitioner to maximize the accuracy of CAD/CAM surgical templates.

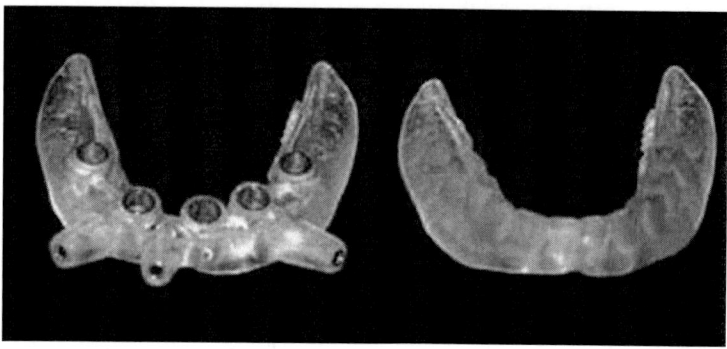

Figure 1. The basic shape of the surgical template is based on the shape of the radiographic template.

First, the correct design of the radiographic guide is fundamental for successful treatment; the geometry of the radiographic guide dictates the shape of the surgical template and is used to simulate tooth position, soft tissue surface, and the edentulous space during a CT scan [1] (Figure 1).

Second, the position of the radiographic template and the position of the surgical template must coincide. Because the intended positions for implant placement are based on the seated position of the radiographic template during the CT scan, the accuracy of implant placement is partly due to the positions of the surgical and radiographic templates being coincident.

Third, a correct centric relation record of the patient must be obtained. Fourth, a correct radiographic and surgical index must be recorded. The practitioner must also be aware of the potential for unintentional volumetric deformation of stereolithographically produced surgical guides compared to the original scanned denture. If volumetric deformation occurs, the surgical guide will lack clinical reliability. In order to avoid deformation, verification of the volumetric congruence is necessary, as is verification of the ISO threshold settings. By checking two sensitive components of guide production, ISO value and volumetric congruence, the practitioner increases the chances of producing an accurate surgical guide. To ensure accurate extraction of the radiographic guide from the cone beam CT image and a precise and stable fit of the surgical template, a calibration device is suggested.

Over the last ten years, analysis of implantology and surgical template-guided implant placement has given insight into important factors to consider and ways to maximize the success of template-guided implant surgery. The practitioner should use implant-planning software during the initial planning for implant placement and prosthesis development. When using a program such as NobelClinician (Nobel Biocare, Zurich), the practitioner should ensure the proper fit of the template, check the long axis with the screw access, and place implants parallel before adjusting angulations. All components should be removed after checking the angulations of the implants and placing anchor pins. Once comprehensive planning is complete, and CAD/CAM templates are ready to be used, several factors must be considered, and necessary steps must be taken to ensure correct template usage:

1. The surgical guide must be accurately placed. The position of the surgical guide should coincide with a radiographic template that is fully seated during the CT scan.
2. Accurate impressions and casts must be made to fabricate the radiographic and surgical templates, and the initial occlusal registration must be accurately recorded to determine the seated template position.
3. Cutouts in the guide should be created over natural tooth abutments to ensure the template is fully seated and is ready to be tried on both the cast and the patient.
4. The practitioner must consider an increased margin of error due to the lack of visibility in a flapless surgical procedure.
5. The practitioner must plan the prefabricated provisional prosthesis for potential interference from the crest of the bone if implants are seated too apically.

Based on accuracy studies, the practitioner should also plan for error at the apex of the implant. While a prefabricated or immediate provisional is a valuable option for guided surgery, it is unnecessary. *Guided surgery* is a technique that can function independently of the type of temporization implemented. Guided implant surgery does not come without its disadvantages. Essential considerations include longer initial treatment times and increased initial setup costs due to template fabrication. Also, because of the bulk of the template and instrumentation, posterior implant placement is often complicated, and additional efforts must be made to ensure proper cooling during osteotomy preparation. Despite the disadvantages of guided implant surgery, the advantages often outweigh the costs. Examination of and reflection upon the evolution of guided surgery has allowed practitioners to improve methods and refine the guided implant surgery procedure. The extent of precision required for anatomical landmarks, implant placement, and restorative procedures allows clinicians to obtain a more predictable result that can lead to increased implant and prosthesis success, longevity, and, ultimately, patient satisfaction [1].

References

[1] Vercruyssen M, Cox C, Naert I, Jacobs R, Teughels W, Quirynen M. Accuracy and patient-centered outcome variables in guided implant surgery: a RCT comparing immediate with delayed loading. *Clin Oral Implants Res.* 2016;27(4):427-32.

Chapter 4

Goals of Guided Implant Surgery

Firstly, and most importantly, to accurately and predictably achieve clinical outcomes transposed from careful diagnostic and pre-surgical planning. Ideally, this should apply to all clinical situations, from single teeth to full arch rehabilitations. It should enable the treatment of challenging sites, such as very narrow ridges. It should reduce the complexity and time of treatment for patients and clinicians. It should ideally enable the pre-construction of a provisional or final prosthesis. It should ideally enable flapless and open flap procedures for implant placement. It should enable complete three-dimensional guidance, i.e., depth, mesio-buccal, and bucco-lingual angulations. Finally, it should become the medico-legal standard of care in most cases and certainly in more complex cases [1].

References

[1] Dunn DB, Guided implant surgery -the new "standard of care?". Australasian Dental Practice. January/February 2009.

Chapter 5

Indications of Guided Implant Surgery

Because of its precision and accuracy, guided surgery may facilitate implant placement. Its many benefits far outweigh the possible objections of time, radiation exposure, and cost. Guided surgery is most beneficial in the following clinical situations [1].

Planning for Three or More Implants in a Row

When three or more implants in a row are planned, concepts of spacing and angulations, parallelism in all dimensions, proximity to anatomic structures, and relationships between implant positions and planned restorations are all significant considerations. CT/CBCT-guided surgery allows for the ideal placement of multiple dental implants according to the planned restoration while considering these issues (Figure 2). Implants can be placed without a flap and immediately loaded.

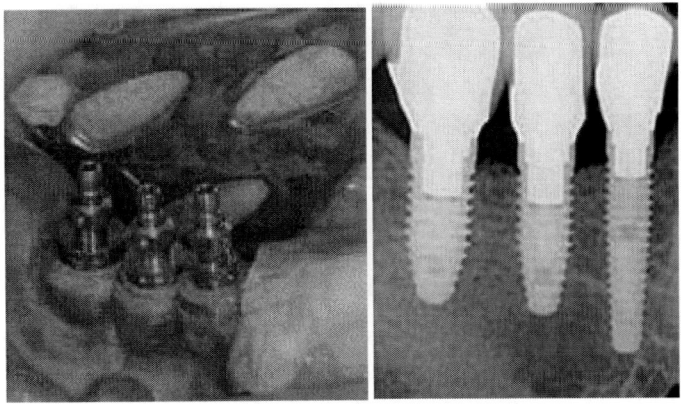

Figure 2. (a) Surgical guide with implants placed attached to implant mounts, (b) three implants in row.

Proximity to Important Anatomic Structures

Panoramic and periapical radiographs are 2-dimensional (2-D) representations of a patient's 3-D anatomy. Differences in radiographic machines and techniques can lead to image distortions such as elongation and shortening of the anatomy. Accurate evaluation and measurement of the relationship between the mental nerve, inferior alveolar nerve (Figure 3), or nasopalatine/incisive nerve and the planned implant position can best be determined and planned by a 3-D evaluation of the anatomy related to the planned restoration. 3,30 Implant placement in patients with a question of nerve or sinus proximity is most accurate using "virtual" treatment planning and placement using CT-generated guides, thus minimizing potential patient morbidity. Technologies such as "all-on-four," designed to maximize the Intra-arch spread of implant platforms while avoiding the mandibular nerve and maxillary sinus, are excellent indications for CT-guided implant surgery.

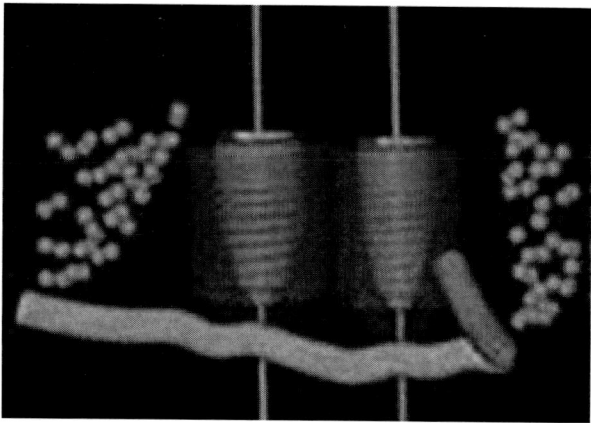

Figure 3. Close proximity to alveolar nerve.

Problems Related to the Proximity of Adjacent Teeth

Surgical dilemmas requiring implant placement in a single location or depth are common. Challenging scenarios frequently necessitate implant placement into tight spaces with minimal bony leeway mesio-distally, bucco-lingually, or both. Adjacent roots may require "threading the needle" with implant placement; this is commonly encountered with congenitally missing teeth.

Limited bone volume often leaves situations where the anatomy dictates where the implant can be placed. All proprietary implant-planning software programs can isolate roots in edentulous areas to aid in accurate implant placement between and adjacent to planned sites. Some software programs use virtual dots or lines to outline the roots.

In contrast, others can alter the software's sensitivity to Hounsfield units or ISO values to remove bone around roots ("segmentation") virtually. These features are beneficial when roots are divergent or convergent or when implants must be placed in tight spaces due to close root proximities. Visualization of adjacent roots allows precise implant positioning in limited mesial-distal spaces. The ideal implant for the specific clinical application can then be selected. Some software programs allow selecting and placing "virtual" stock and custom abutments.

Questionable Bone Volume

In cases involving limited bone volume, including deficient width, height, or unusual bony contours, the anatomy often dictates where an implant can be placed—usually in one location only. A CT or CBCT evaluation of the site can lead to decisions to perform preparatory grafting procedures. Three-dimensional evaluation of a grafted site provides valuable information on the amount and location of the grafted bone volume, allowing for accurate implant placement. If guided implant placement is planned, a second CT or CBCT may occasionally be indicated after grafting. In extraction or immediate implant placement patients, concavities can be found in the bone apical to the tooth to be extracted. Fenestrations and perforations can occur if this is not recognized preoperatively. In the anterior maxilla, the thickness of the palatal bone can be instrumental in determining whether an extraction with immediate implant placement can be accomplished with good primary stability.

Implant Position: Critical to the Restoration

Some of the most complex restorative and surgical patients treated in implant dentistry involve single and multiple implants in the esthetic zone. Thicknesses of crestal and buccal soft tissues and buccal and palatal cortical plates, buccal-lingual ridge dimensions, proximity to adjacent teeth, implant-to-root relationships, gingival and papilla support and contours, gingival exposure, smile lines, and implant angulations and emergence are a few of the many complex considerations. An important prosthetic consideration is knowledge of the appropriate implant position based on the type of restoration planned (cement- or screw-retained). Slight variations in implant positions can lead to complex restorative dilemmas. Accurate and predictable implant positioning using guided implant planning and placement can be critical to the esthetic and functional success of the restoration (Figure 4) [2].

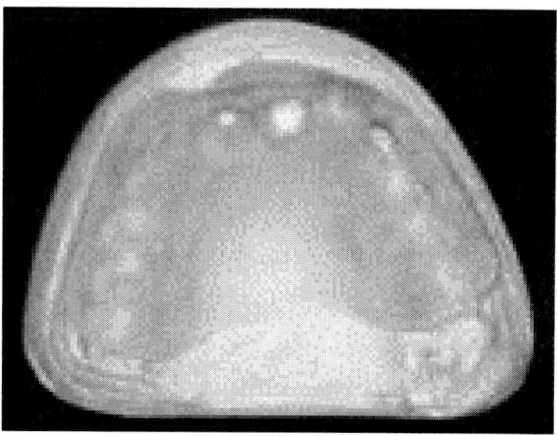

Figure 4. Surgical guide fabricated from virtual plan.

References

[1] Norkin FJ, Ganeles J, Zfaz S, Modares A. Assessing image-guided implant surgery in today's clinical practice. *Compend Contin Educ Dent*. 2013;34(10):747-50.

[2] Van Assche N, Vercruyssen M, Coucke W, Teughels W, Jacobs R, Quirynen M. Accuracy of computer-aided implant placement. *Clin Oral Implants Res*. 2012;23 Suppl 6:112-23.

Chapter 6

Advantages of Guided Implant Surgery

There are many advantages to guided implant surgery, and these relate to the leading three "players" in the relationship: the patient, the practitioner(s), and the dental technician. For the patient, guided surgery (with experienced operators) does offer the ability to achieve the highest level of diagnosis utilizing the various software planning programs available today and, from this planning, develop a treatment plan with the placement of implants (and ultimately the definitive prosthesis) undertaken predictably and in strict accordance with this treatment plan. In the absence of other variables (the validity of the diagnosis and treatment plan, surgical skill and experience, the skill of the laboratory technician, etc.), patients can have more predictable treatment, resulting in a higher level of safety and, ultimately, the desired aesthetic and functional outcome.

In many cases, especially in flapless or "blind techniques," this can decrease swelling, bleeding, and discomfort. The number of procedures and hence the time requirement (for the patient) can be decreased significantly, and in many instances, costs can also be reduced. For the clinician, the advantages of guided surgery are compelling, especially for the "single operator." Various advanced software planning systems currently facilitate accurate diagnosis and treatment planning, such as NobelGuide, SimPlant, and Med 3-D. These programs are utilized to design surgical templates based on the planning process. However, all systems have various pros and cons, and not all systems achieve the same level of accuracy or control.

By far, the most significant advantage for the clinician is the ability to visualize their patient's hard and soft tissue anatomy and "test" their proposed treatment plan and various options within this plan before any intervention is undertaken. While in most cases, it enables the determination of an appropriate treatment plan, in others, it may eliminate that patient from initial treatment and determine the need for either or both hard and soft tissue grafting prior to future implant treatment. Further, it enables an appropriate dialogue with the patient, describing their proposed treatment plan in detail, including risk assessment and the ability to outline the options for treatment or identify any compromising factors. Again, predictability is the key, and the ability to minimize unknowns and operator variables is very significant.

While there is undoubtedly an increased time requirement in the diagnostic work-up and the computer planning and assessment stages for the clinician, there is a significant potential for savings in the context of clinical time, which is a critical issue for most. Complex cases, such as narrow ridges and minimal bone above the inferior alveolar nerve (IAN), nasal or sinus floors, "all on four" techniques utilizing angled distal fixtures to avoid either the maxillary sinus or the IAN, in mandibular cases, "closed or blind" placement of Zygomaticus implants, narrow mesiodistal spaces with close root proximity, and flapless procedures, are but some of the examples where guided surgery is of enormous benefit.

The ability to construct a provisional or definitive prosthesis before implant placement and have confidence that the prosthesis, with appropriate surgical skills, can be placed at the time of surgery is certainly of benefit. However, at this stage, only the NobelGuide system (Nobel Biocare) with trustworthy three-dimensional guidance and the placement of the implants through the surgical template, including depth control and utilizing their specific "guided abutment" to accommodate any minor discrepancies, can achieve this reality. However, the author believes most immediately placed restorations should be provisional only, and immediate function should only be utilized when the appropriate criteria have been met.

The ability to test the prosthetic design with provisional restorations prior to definitive restorations provides the opportunity to make changes, have try-in procedures, accommodate any soft tissue changes following implant placement, and more readily confirm successful osseointegration prior to embarking on expensive laboratory procedures. Having a provisional prosthesis pre-constructed and inserted on the same day of surgery or the next day is a significant advantage and an excellent motivator for patients. Many practitioners, especially with more complex cases, are often "caught" with increased costs at the laboratory level that were initially unforeseen. Guided surgery, enabling the achievement of the predetermined prosthetic plan, minimizes the risks of more complicated technical procedures being required to accommodate issues such as angulation issues, minimal soft tissue dimensions, and too close proximity of implants [1].

References

[1] Dunn DB. Guided implant surgery - The new "standard of care?" *Australasian Dental Practice*. 2009 January/February 2009.

Chapter 7

Disadvantages of Guided Implant Surgery

- An expensive CT machine is necessary.
- The patient's bone situation cannot be assessed when doing flapless surgery.
- The surgery planning time takes longer.
- The user must learn the planning software.
- Any unexpected situations during surgery are unmanageable.
- Surgical kits and surgical templates must be purchased.

Chapter 8

Guided Implant Surgery Systems

There are currently three major guided surgery systems available on the local market: NobelGuide (Nobel Biocare); SimPlant (Materialise, available through Tomatic); and Med 3-D AG (available through Alphabond). It is important to state unequivocally that guided surgery, especially when combined with immediate loading, is no "slam dunk" and should only be undertaken by clinicians with appropriate training and surgical and restorative experience. The author firmly believes that, at present, these systems are all being advertised and promoted as "entry-level" technology for inexperienced users with minimal training, but this can only lead to complications and, most importantly, unhappy patients. This technology is no substitute for surgical or prosthodontic experience, and certainly not the "panacea of all ills" when it comes to implant treatment!

Here is a brief overview of each:

- SimPlant and Med 3-D can utilize most implant brands today, whereas NobelGuide is restricted to Nobel Biocare implants.
- All three systems have good to excellent 3-dimensional planning.
- All three systems can utilize either CT or cone beam scans.
- NobelGuide and Med 3-D utilize raw DICOM data. SimPlant requires DICOM files to be "processed" for a fee before using the software unless the clinician has invested in the highest-level "PRO" software.
- A double-scan technique (where the patient and template are scanned together and then the template is scanned separately) is preferable to avoid artefacts in the scans. NobelGuide is the only system utilizing a double-scan.
- The radiographic template design is critical, as is its stabilization while radiographic imaging is undertaken. The NobelGuide protocol includes the use of an occlusal index to stabilize and maintain the orientation of the radiographic template while scanning procedures are The other systems utilize a passively seated template with no stabilization. All systems are at risk of errors with movements or

incorrect positioning of the radiographic template at the time of the scanning procedures.
- The stabilization of the surgical template is also critical. The NobelGuide system achieves this by utilizing anchor pins, which are 1.5-mm-diameter lateral stabilizing pins designed at the planning stage and incorporated into the template. No other system has this. This is especially important in unbounded saddles and, Obviously, in fully edentulous situations. SimPlant does have optional 2mm retention screws to stabilize the template at the time of surgery.
- The SimPlant "safe" system provides accurate 3-dimensional control and implant placement through the template; however, it is restricted to external hex implants only and to diameters between 75 mm and 4.1 mm.
- The Med 3-D system is mainly utilized with a single 2 mm pilot hole sleeve; however, several templates can be constructed with other diameter sleeves. Implant placement is not undertaken through the template.
- SimPlant typically provides three templates with varying diameter sleeves according to practitioner preference. However, this can complicate issues with multiple implants of varying SimPlant "turnaround time" from the complex model and radiographic template being sent to the production facility in Belgium, which is approximately two weeks. Med 3-D utilizes the fabrication and conversion of the radiographic template to a surgical template. This usually takes approximately one week and is undertaken with a designated local dental laboratory (with the "Hexapod" device required for conversion). The NobelGuide delivery time from receipt of electronic data to receipt of the surgical template is approximately ten days.
- NobelGuide can be used with either computer-based planning or with model-based SimPlant requires the model and template to be sent to Belgium for template fabrication, of which 90% to 95% are manufactured. Med 3-D utilizes the modification of the radiographic template and is converted "in-house" by the designated local laboratory. The NobelGuide planning data is sent via the internet, with the fabrication of the template by the stereolithographic process in either the US or Sweden.
- Med 3-D utilizes implant company drilling and placement equipment per the selected implant type. The operator provides all componentry

for use with Med 3-D, apart from the sleeves in the template; however, the practitioner needs to account for the guide dimensions with their drilling protocols. SimPlant provides up to three diameters of sleeves in their "Surgi-guides," one per guide, but has no depth control for implant placement (apart from their "SAFE" system, but with restrictions).

- The SimPlant "SAFE" system has its "own" drilling and implant carrier. A single template is used with interchangeable sleeves. Only two drills for 3.75 mm and 4.1 mm diameter external hex implants are used. This may cause difficulties with the drilling protocol for different bone types and densities.
- SimPlant also now has "Navigator" for the 3i-Biomet implant system and "Facilitate" for all Astra "Osseospeed" The "Navigator" system is a "rebadged" SimPlant that enables the use of "CERTAIN" style 3i-Biomet parallel-walled, internal connection implants of all diameters. Implants are inserted through the template, giving proper 3D control. Prosthetic abutment options are available for "Certain implants" to enable early or immediate loading. Similar to "Navigator," Astra also now has a "rebadged" SimPlant called "Facilitate." Materialize (SimPlant) can also now produce a NobelGuide template "clone" compatible with NobelGuide drilling componentry and Guide sleeves. Dentsply will soon release its guided surgery system, also based on the Materialize platform, for its Friadent range of implants, called "Expertease."
- NobelGuide has a complete system with interchangeable drilling guides (with a single template) specific to the implant type and diameter, including fixture placement through the template and vertical control of both the implant osteotomy and the implant. Further, when the template is ordered, all components relevant to the case (including laboratory needs) are assembled and available for order simultaneously. This eliminates the problem of ordering errors and componentry being "missed."
- SimPlant and Med 3-D templates can be bone, soft tissue, or tooth-supported, using flapless or flap techniques. Nobel Guide is tooth and/or soft-tissue-supported, designed primarily for a flapless However. The templates can be utilized with a technique variation for immediate and flap procedures.
- The NobelGuide template design utilizes extended flanges, which may create difficulties with high lip line smiles and assessing lip

support. Patients may also be required to wear a removable prosthesis for approximately six months while teeth are removed, and healing occurs. Further, some operators are skilled with immediate placement and loading and thus can reduce treatment time and eliminate the removable prosthesis stage in treatment, but may see this step as a hindrance or unnecessary.

- The implant placement sequence and torque utilized are also critical factors in all systems concerning three-dimensional implant placement accuracy, especially with the torquing or tipping of the template with a free-end saddle or in some fully edentulous cases such as with mandible.
- All systems enable the treatment of complex cases such as thin ridges or critical angulation placements.
- There is a need for approximately 45 to 50 mm of opening for most guided componentry and the corresponding drilling. This equates to approximately 10 mm of increased drill lengths compared to "normal." This may restrict the use of this technology in some instances. However, with SimPlant, the template's and sleeves' vertical dimensions can be changed, especially in difficult vertical spaces such as posterior situations. According to planning, the "Navigator" system uses integrated depth stops of various dimensions. In contrast, the "Facilitate" system uses disposable drills on a case-by-case basis with integrated depth stops or standard drills. NobelGuide utilizes built-in drill stops with its tapered range of implants and adjustable drill stops for its parallel-walled implant options.
- There is a difficulty with partially edentulous cases with narrow mesio-distal dimensions to enable room for the template and drill sleeve componentry. This may readily be seen in lower anterior cases or, alternatively, in maxillary central or lateral.
- There is a tendency to "drill to prescription" rather than appreciate the "feel" of the bone density in the osteotomy preparation, often leading to overpreparation. Hence, loss of primary stability, especially in inexperienced Again, is relevant to all systems, especially NobelGuide and SimPlant Safe (including Navigator and Facilitate).
- In the placement of implants through the template, there is also a tendency to over-torque the implants, effectively compromising primary stability by "pulling the implant" through the bone on tightening. Again, this is specific to systems where the implants are

placed through the template, e.g., NobelGuide and SimPlant Safe (including Navigator and Facilitate).
- The use of a flapless approach in treatment potentially loses some attached soft tissue dimension, and this may be especially relevant and difficult to control in mandibular However, with appropriate planning and controls, a flapless approach, in the indicated cases, offers greater predictability, minimal soft tissue changes, and considerably less discomfort for the patient. SimPlant "Surgi-guides" and "Safe" systems (including Navigator and Facilitate), as well as Med 3-D, require a "pick-up" impression or registration of a prefabricated prosthesis and then a laboratory step to complete the prosthesis. "Facilitate" has some provisional abutment componentry enabling early or immediate loading.
- NobelGuide has a "guided abutment," which, along with the ability to place the implant through the template, enables the insertion of the provisional (or indeed definitive) restoration at the time of implant placement to achieve true immediate However, in the author's opinion, in the majority of cases, a preconstructed provisional prosthesis can be "picked up" with temporary or definitive abutments and added to the prosthesis in a simple laboratory procedure on the same day or overnight at worst. This will provide the most accurate solution and improve the health of the epithelial cuff around the abutment.
- No five-year multicenter studies published on guided implant surgery are available as of yet. Henry P. J. et al. published a 94.1% survival rate in partially edentulous cases, which compares favourably with his multicenter partially edentulous jaw study.
- Most importantly, all three systems enable the use of the planning software as a planning tool only, all the way through to the construction and use of surgical templates constructed from the computerized treatment plan [1].

References

[1] Dunn DB. Guided implant surgery - The new "standard of care?" *Australasian Dental Practice*. 2009 January/February 2009.

Chapter 9

Guided Surgical Templates

The use of a transfer device is essential to establish logical continuity between diagnosis, prosthetic planning, and surgical phases. After the presurgical restorative appointments, the restoring dentist fabricates the surgical guide template once the final prosthetic design, occlusal scheme, implant location, size, and angulation have been determined. The surgical template dictates the implant body placement that offers the best combination of (1) support for the repetitive forces of occlusion, (2) esthetics and (3) hygiene requirements. A well-developed plan should be transferred precisely, leaving little room for decision during surgery. Several methods of fabricating the surgical template are available. The requirements are more relevant than the options for fabrication. The template should be stable and rigid when in the correct position. If the arch being treated has remaining teeth, the template should fit over or around enough teeth to stabilize it in position. (Figure 5).

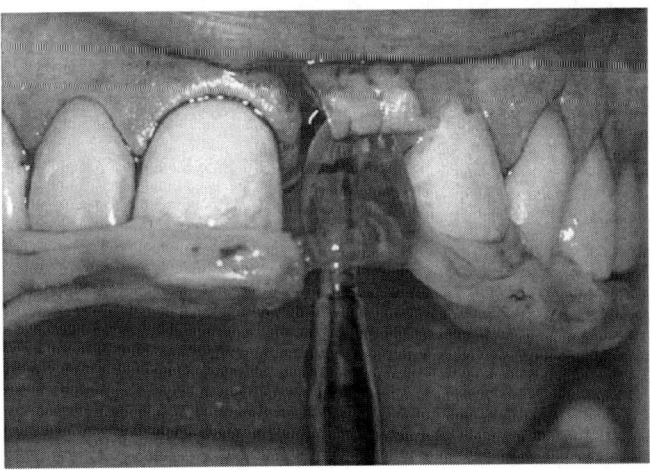

Figure 5. Templates for the anterior regions of the mouth.

When no remaining teeth are present, the template should extend onto unreflected soft tissue regions (i.e., the palate and tuberosities in the maxilla or the retromolar pads in the mandible). This way, the template may be used after the soft tissues have been removed from the implant site [1].

The Glossary of Prosthodontic Terms (GPT) defines a surgical template as a guide to assist in the proper surgical placement and angulation of dental implants. It enables prediction and minimally invasive surgery. The main objective of the surgical template is to direct the implant drilling system and provide accurate placement of the implant according to the surgical treatment plan. Customized conventional radiographic or computer-image-guided surgical templates have become the treatment of choice. A surgical guide consists of two components: The guiding cylinders and the contact surface. The contact surface fits either on an element of a patient's gums or jaw (i.e., the bone or the teeth). A cylinder within the drill guides helps transfer the drill to its exact location and orientation. The implant must be placed so that the bottom and sides are fully covered by bone or bone-replacement material. Care should be taken not to damage any neighbouring anatomic structures. These are, in particular, the mandibular nerve in the mandible, the Schneiderian membrane of the maxillary sinus in the maxilla, and also the roots of adjacent teeth. Thirdly, the implant's position must be compatible with the intended final prosthodontic restoration [2].

The dentist should determine the ideal angulation for implant insertion on the diagnostic wax-up, and the template should relate to this position during surgery. This requires at least two reference points for each implant. The surgical guide must be elevated above the edentulous bone for that purpose. The distance between the two points located respectively on the occlusal surface (central fossa or incisal edge) of the planned abutment crown and the crest of the ridge is about 8 mm. As a result, these two points of reference can be joined by a line representing the path of ideal implant insertion. The ideal angulation is perpendicular to the occlusal plane and parallel to the most anterior abutment (natural or implant) joined to the implant. Other ideal requirements of the surgical template include size, surgical asepsis, transparency, and the ability to revise the template as indicated. The template should not be bulky, difficult to insert, or obscure surrounding surgical landmarks. The surgical template must not contaminate a surgical field during bone grafts or implant placement; it should also be transparent and allow easy access for the surgeon and the assistant. Consideration of which side of the arch is being treated, where the surgeon and assistant will be seated, and whether the surgeon is right- or left-handed is recommended. In this way, the bony ridge and drills can be more easily visualized when the template is in place, and the assistant can position the irrigation without blocking the surgical view. The surgical template should relate to the ideal facial contour.

Many edentulous ridges have lost facial bone, and the template can assist in determining the amount of augmentation required for implant placement or support of the lips and face. The surgical template may be used for a bone graft, and later the same template may be used for the insertion of implants and again for implant uncover. A study template facilitates sterilization and is used for several procedures. To construct a surgical guide, modification of the radiographic guide is often possible if an ideal wax-up of the teeth is used as a template for the radiographic guide. Ideal tooth position is already present, and enlargement of the access hole and a buccal or lingual opening is easily achieved. When the long axis of the teeth is visible and can be maintained after verifying bone availability, then enlargement of the long axis channel guarantees accurate implant guidance.

An easy method to fabricate a surgical guide is using a modified version of Preston's clear splint to diagnose tooth contours, position, and occlusal form. The diagnostic wax-up is completed to preview the tooth size, position, contour, and occlusion in the edentulous regions where implants will be inserted. No selective grinding or modification is performed on teeth that have not been altered before surgery; otherwise, the templates will not fit correctly in the mouth. A full-arch, irreversible hydrocolloid impression is made of the diagnostic wax-up and poured into dental stone. On the duplicate cast of the wax-up teeth, a vacuum acrylic shell (0.060 to 0.080 inch) is pressed and trimmed to fit over the teeth and gingival contours of the buccal aspect of the ridge. If no natural teeth remain, the posterior portion of the template should be maintained and cover the retromolar pads, tuberosities, and palate to aid in positioning. The occlusal surface is trimmed over the ideal and optional implant sites, maintaining the surgical template's facial and facio-occlusal line angles (Figure 6).

A black line is then drawn on the template with a marker to indicate the centre of each implant and the desired angulation. This provides maximum freedom for implant placement while communicating the ideal tooth position and angulation during surgery. A surgical guide template with 2-mm holes through the occlusal surface of a denture tooth is too limiting for the surgeon, although it precisely identifies the ideal implant placement. While the template is in position, the crest of the edentulous ridge should be visible to avoid stripping the facial plate of bone during the osteotomy. The vacuum form may be fabricated from the existing removable prosthesis in the edentulous arch if within accepted guidelines.

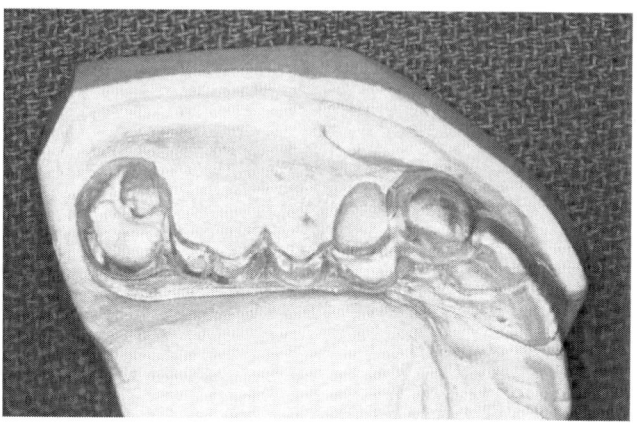

Figure 6. The template is trimmed in the edentulous sites to indicate the teeth position.

A soft tissue liner may then be added to the tuberosity, retromolar pad regions, and other soft tissue areas not involved in the surgery. Acrylic resin is then added over the occlusal portion of the template, where no implants are planned. The patient then occludes this index after using petroleum jelly over the opposing teeth. In this manner, the template can be correctly positioned over the edentulous ridge during surgery once the tissue is removed. Otherwise, a template position is likely set too far forward or off to one side (Figure 7).

A surgical template for the complete edentulous arch may also engage the occlusal aspect of the opposing teeth. The following are the fabrication steps on the edentulous cast mounted against the opposing dentition at the proper final occlusal vertical dimension and occlusal relationships:

1. A full wax-up of the missing teeth in the edentulous regions is performed. A hole is prepared through the middle of the central fossa of each future posterior abutment tooth and the incisal edge position of the anterior.
2. On the stone model, each site chosen is drilled to a depth corresponding to the approximate soft tissue thickness measured on a panoramic radiograph (approximately 2 to 3 mm). An orthodontic wire is passed through the teeth and into the holes. This allows each

pin of the template to contact the bone once the tissue is reflected during the surgery without modifying the occlusal vertical dimension and consequently the emergence position of the A small loop is made at the other end of the wire to create a retention form. The wire should approach the opposing arch within 1 to 3 mm (Figure 8).

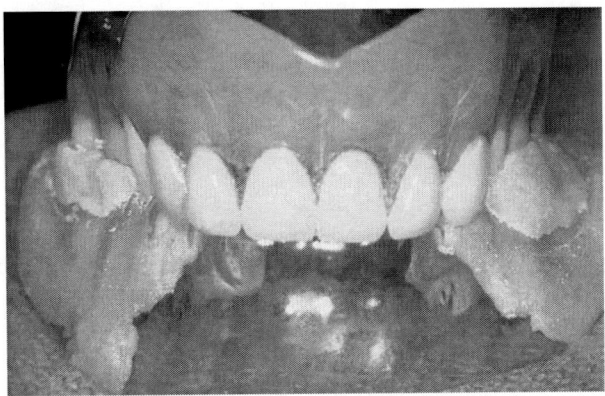

Figure 7. A soft tissue liner is added in the area that will not be reflected during surgery.

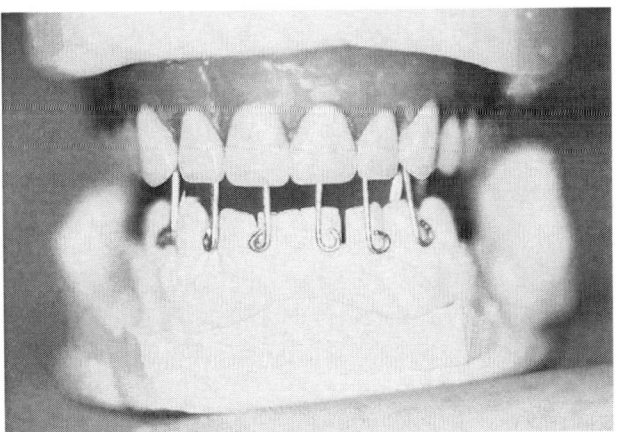

Figure 8. A Laney-Poitras template for the edentulous arch provides complete surgical access.

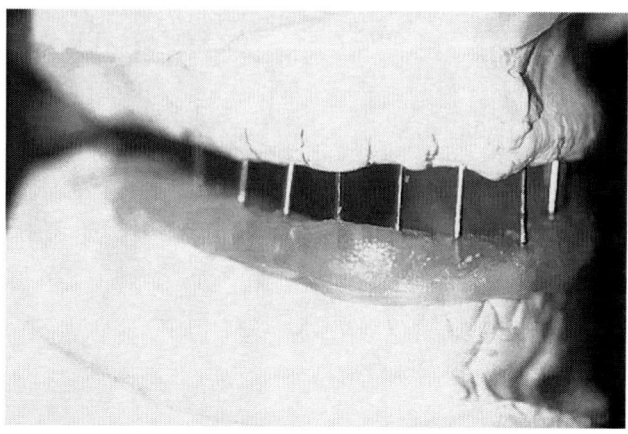

Figure 9. The wires representing each potential implant site and angulation are incorporated into an acrylic index of the opposing arch.

3. On the antagonist model painted with a separator, an acrylic resin template is built on the occlusal that embeds the retention loops of the indicator pins. Each pin must be embedded entirely in the acrylic at the proper centric and vertical relationships (Figure 9).

Once the soft tissue is reflected, the template is positioned over the teeth of the opposing arch. The patient may occlude the pins, and each one determines the ideal centre position of the teeth (Figures 10, 11). A pilot drill can be used to mark each implant's body position. The angulation of the osteotomy can also be determined with the template. The surgical guide quickly determines the implant position, yet the surgeon can have the patient's mouth open and drill into the bone with complete access and vision. This template may also be used with a panoramic radiograph before surgery to determine vertical magnificence or horizontal distortion. The template may also be used at stage II uncover to find the position of each implant when soft tissue carving for fixed prosthesis type 1 (FP-1).

Restorations are indicated rather than complete removal of the tissue. The FP-1 and FP-2 restorations require ideal implant placement. The ideal implant position allows the placement of a straight abutment directly under the incisal edge of the final crown for a cemented prosthesis. For screw-retained prostheses, the implant should emerge toward the cingulum of the anterior tooth so that the access hole does not affect the esthetics.

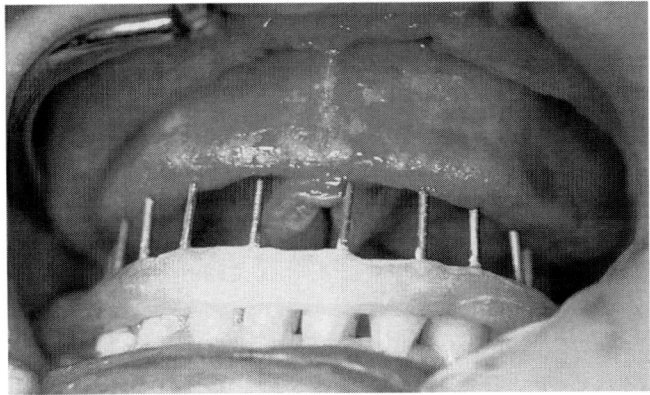

Figure 10. Template is seated on the opposing arch and indicates the position and angulation of each implant.

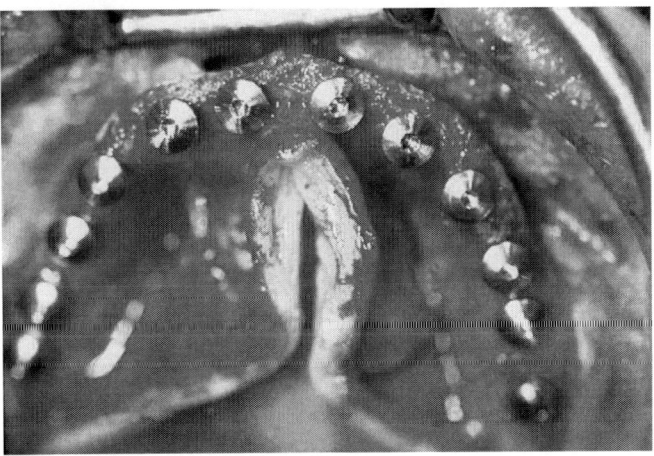

Figure 11. Implants are inserted into the maxilla in the appropriate positions.

In an FP-3 restoration, the mesiodistal position of implant abutments may be placed without regard to the actual position of the crowns because the soft tissue replacement region separates the crowns from the implant abutment.

An implant adjacent to a natural tooth should remain 1.5 to 2 mm away from the interproximal cement-enamel junction (CEJ) in esthetic regions where the contour of the interdental papilla is a determining factor. Therefore, the pilot hole should be almost 4 mm from the natural tooth to place a 4.1-mm-diameter implant at the crest module. This requires at least a 7-mm mesio-distal space. In unesthetic regions, where the interdental papilla is not as critical, an implant placed at least 1.5 mm away from an adjacent tooth minimizes the risk of surgical error and provides easier access for hygiene and long-term maintenance. A maxillary anterior implant placed for an FP-1 restoration requires careful pretreatment planning and precise implant placement. The incisal edge of the final crown, emergence prominence, and labial cervical position are related to implant position. The treatment plan for an implant in the maxillary first premolar position must reflect careful consideration for the angulation of a natural canine when present. The 11-degree average distal inclination and distal curvature of the canine root bring the apex of the root into the first premolar implant area. Therefore, the implant should be angled to follow the root of the canine and prevent contact with or perforation of the natural root. A shorter implant is often indicated, especially when a second premolar is also present [3].

References

[1] D'Souza KM, Aras MA. Types of implant surgical guides in dentistry: a review. *J Oral Implantol*. 2012 Oct;38(5):643-52

[2] Rohit Shah. Guided implant surgery. *Int Educ Res J*. 2017;3(11).

[3] Kathleen Manuela D'Souza. Types of Implant Surgical Guides in Dentistry: AReview. *Journal of Oral Implantology*. 2012; 13(5).

Chapter 10

Types of Surgical Templates

Three types of surgical guides can be fabricated for precise guided implant placement:

- *Teeth-supported*
  These guides are fabricated for partially edentulous patients using teeth as support for the guide.
- *Mucosa-supported*
  These guides are fabricated for completely edentulous patients whose mucosa supports the guide. Inter-arch records are made to determine the vertical dimension. These guides are secured during surgery with the help of fixation screws to prevent movement of the guide.
- *Bone-supported*
  These guides can be used in partially or wholly edentulous patients, but primarily in patients with atrophied mucosa that prevents proper seating of the guide. A full-thickness flap is raised, exposing the bone to seat the guide [1].

Table 1. Implant Planing systems

Manufacturer	Guided surgery software
Nobel	Nobelguide
Mayerialised dental	SimPlant
Denrsply	Facilitate (Astratech)
Biodenta	Bioguide
3Sgape	Implant studio
Straumann	Codiagnostix
Sirona	Implant 3D (galileos)

Following the completion of implant planning in the Invivo software, Anatomage fabricates the surgical guide known as the Anatomage Guide. The following types of templates are currently available for the Anatomage guide:

- Tooth-supported
- Mucosa-supported
- Bone-supported reduction and implant surgical guides (mandible only)

Universal Master Sleeves

The anatomage guide controls the trajectory and osteotomy depth through the master sleeve integrated into the acrylic drill guide template. A unique feature of the Anatomage Guide is the universal master sleeve that allows a clinician to insert any implant that uses a parallel drilling protocol, such as Straumann Bone Level, Nobel Active/Speedy, Dentsply AstraTech, and Zest Locator Overdenture Implants (LODI). The handle and drill kits accommodate narrow sleeves (3.1mm), regular sleeves (4.1mm), and wide sleeves (5.1mm), and the drill kit includes 21mm and 26mm universal drills (Figure 12).

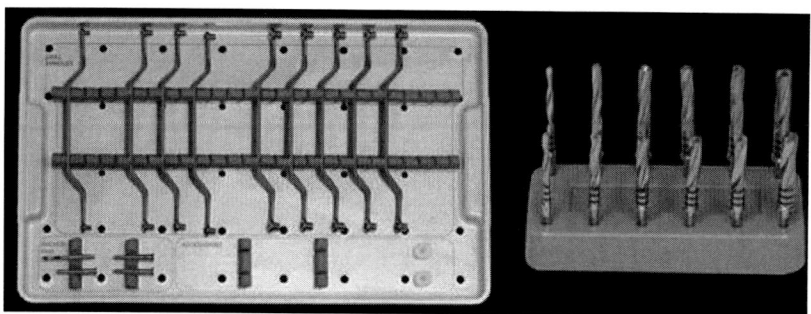

Figure 12. Universal Anatomage Guide drills and handles allow for osteotomy preparation for multiple systems.

The universal kit allows complete osteotomy preparation except for drill tapping and final implant insertion (partially guided); these procedures should be performed without the guide in the mouth. Suppose a tapered implant drilling protocol is required. In that case, universal drills should be used until the last drill size, and the final tapered drill in the manufacturer's kit should be used to prepare the final osteotomy. Raising or lowering the sleeve position in relation to the controls mentioned above for implant depth while tilting the master sleeves in relation to teeth, mucosa, or bone controls implant trajectory. When using a universal kit, the clinician must know the surgical drilling protocol for the respective implant. For example, if a

3.5 mm x 11.5 mm Nobel Replace implant were to be placed, the universal drilling protocol would be a guided universal 2.0 mm drill, followed by a guided universal 2.8 mm drill, and finally, a non-guided Nobel tapered 3.5 mm x 13mm drill.

Manufacturer-Specific Master Sleeves

If preferred, Anatomage can also fabricate guides with manufacturer-specific master sleeves for the following systems:

Table 2. Specific master sleeves

Nobel Guide	Zimmer
3i Navigator	Straumann
Camlog	Implant Direct

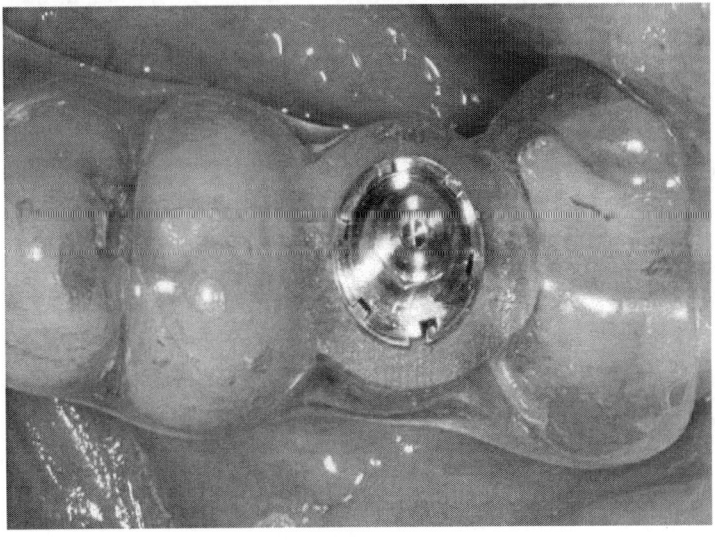

Figure 13. Manufacturer specific master sleeve with a universal guide allows for a fully-guided implant surgical procedure.

Manufacturer-specific master sleeves allow whole trajectory and depth control, guided drill taps, and guided implant insertion (Figure 13). However, fully guided implant insertion capability with an anatomy guide is currently available only for NobelBiocare, 3i, and Camlog implant systems. Complete implant guidance may be less of an issue for clinicians who routinely use guided surgery to place implants without immediate provisional restorations prefabricated in the laboratory. If a clinician wishes to have a provisional restoration prefabricated to be delivered on the day of implant insertion, fully guided implant placement may be necessary.

Universal Templates (Pilot Surgiguide, Universal Surgiguide)

Pilot SurgiTemplates control initial trajectory and osteotomy depth through the master sleeve integrated into the acrylic drill guide template. The pilot surgical guide provides drill guidance and depth control for the pilot drill only, which is typically 2.0 mm in diameter. Once the pilot osteotomy is performed, the guide is removed, and the remainder of the drilling and implant placement is performed without the guide's assistance. This guide is recommended for experienced users who want guidance during the initial drilling step. Universal SurgiTemplates control the full trajectory and osteotomy depth through the master sleeve.

The universal guide allows for comprehensive drilling guidance from pilot to final drills; however, this depends on the implant system used. If an implant is being placed that requires a tapered drilling protocol (Nobel Replace or 3i Tapered Certain), the last drill must be performed without the assistance of the guide. Complete osteotomy can be performed entirely through the guide for cylindrical drilling protocol implants (Nobel Active, 3i Parallel, and Implant Direct Legacy). After the completion of the drilling protocol, the guide is removed, and the implant is placed without the assistance of the guide. A drill and handle kit from the manufacturer is available for use by either the pilot or universal SurgiGuide. Available in three diameters (1.95, 2.75, and 3.15 mm) and six lengths (15, 18, 20, 23, 25, and 28 mm), drills are available from the manufacturer (SurgiGuideLongStop Drills, Materialise NV) for use in the pilot and universal templates (Figure 14).

Types of Surgical Templates

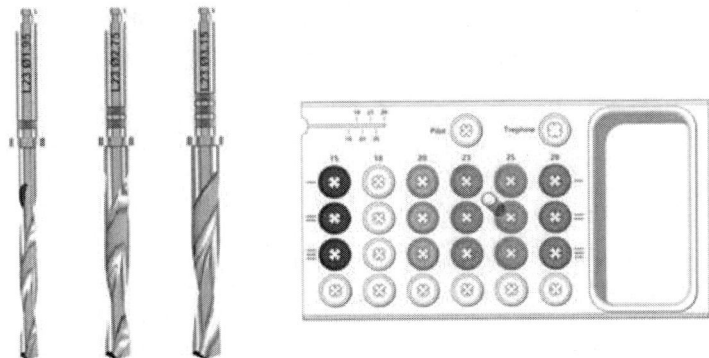

Figure 14. Universal drills for the Simplant SurgiGuide system allows for the initial osteotomy preparation.

Manufacturer-Specific Guide (SAFE SurgiGuide)

If preferred, Materialise can also fabricate a guide with manufacturer-specific master sleeves for the following systems:

Table 3. Manufacturer specific guide

AstraTech Facilitate	Camlog
3i Navigator	Straumann Safe
Nobel Guide	Friadent Expertease
	Zimmer

SAFE SurgiTemplates allow for full trajectory and depth control, guided drill taps, and guided implant insertion. This method allows for fully guided implant insertion; however, fully guided implant insertion capability is currently available only for Nobel, 3i, Camlog, and AstraTech. Zimmer, Straummann, and Friadent implants can be placed through the guide. However, the guide will not fully control the guidance depth, and turn of the implant Bone-supported templates are available with the option of a stereolithographic maxilla or mandible [2] (Figure 15).

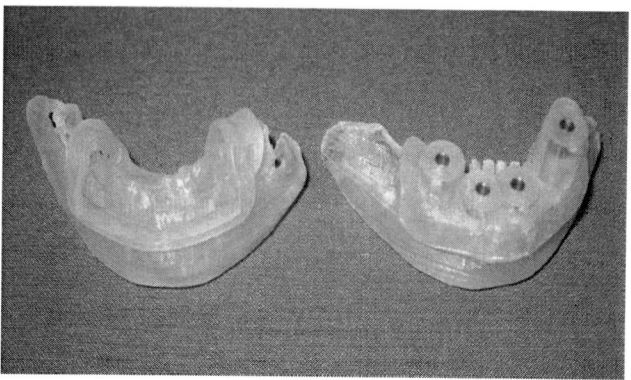

Figure 15. Stereolithographic mandibles illustrating a bone reduction and an implant surgical guide.

Customized Conventional Radiographic Surgical Template:

The surgical template uses a conventional radiographic method and requires a thorough radiographic examination and proper diagnosis of the bony. Panoramic radiography is still the standard for the planning of implants. However, precise measurement of the bone architecture is impossible because OPGs have a magnification factor that is not always uniform. Therefore, a better assessment of the bone dimensions in panoramic radiographs is made by determining the magnification factor. Conventional dental panoramic radiography and plain film radiography are usually performed with the patient wearing a radiographic template with integrated metal spheres or rods, sleeves, and guide posts at the position of the wax. Based on the magnification factor and the known dimensions of the metal, the depth and dimensions of the implants are planned. The implant placement planning is guided by the quality and quantity of bone and the position of the teeth for esthetics and phonetics.

Fabrication Process

Several types of surgical guides have been reported in the literature. Some are designed for the placement of a single implant, while other reports present designs for implant-fixed partial dentures, multiple single implants, and implant-retained overdentures. Some of the most commonly used techniques are mentioned briefly here.

Diagnostic casts of the dental arches are made from irreversible hydrocolloid impressions. A diagnostic wax-up of the proposed case of an implant-supported FPD is done. A silicone impression of the cast with the waxed FPD is made as a mould. A clear, chemically activated acrylic resin is poured into the mould space and cured. Access holes are made according to information obtained from the cast model for the initial surgical drill. Stainless steel guide sleeves of uniform length are cut, placed in access holes, and cured. 8 Another method to prepare a radiographic guide is to use vacuum-formed templates. After the diagnostic waxing of the final restoration is completed, duplication is made, and a cast is poured. The vacuum-formed template fabricated is placed over the cast, and the edentulous space is filled with radio-opaque material (Barium sulfate, lead strip, gutta-percha). 9 In another method, two vacuum-formed templates are used, one over the blocked-out diagnostic cast and the other over the duplicate cast of the diagnostic wax, and a clear plastic sheet is made. Both templates are returned to the unaltered diagnostic cast. The edges of the two templates are trimmed to make them coincide. The diagnostic wax template is removed and filled with clear orthodontic resin or radio-opaque material. The filled template is placed over the template of the unaltered diagnostic cast. Holes are made according to information obtained from the radiograph for the placement of implants, followed by the placement of drill guides.

The milling technique is accurate and employs parallel holes in the surgical guide. This technique needs the aid of a conventional dental surveyor. All conventionally made radiographic guides can be converted to accurate surgical guides utilizing this milling technique. The limitation of this technique is that it requires special equipment that is not commonly available in private dental practices. In addition, the practitioner needs a certain amount of experience and knowledge to operate this machine properly. However, panoramic radiography, which is still the standard and widely used, has diagnostic limitations such as expansion and distortion, setting error, positional artefacts, and no information regarding the dimension of bone in the bucco-lingual direction. Further, these surgical templates are fabricated on dental casts, which are rigid, non-functional surfaces without knowledge of the underlying soft tissue resiliency and bone topography. Anatomical landmarks are not precisely located; they do not show the lingual blood vessels, and approaches are always two-dimensional. So, there are more chances of malpositioning the implants during placement, resulting in less stability during surgery. The success of the outcome always depends on the clinician's skill, which requires more chair time, leading to stress for the dentist and patient. Although conventional surgical templates will allow the placement of implant guides, they do not provide exact 3D guidance.

Computer-Generated Surgical Template

Computer-generated surgical templates have evolved to overcome the limitations associated with conventional radiographic surgical templates. A computer-generated surgical guide links our treatment plan and surgery by accurately transferring the simulated plan to the surgical site. This surgical guide is made using the stereolithography process and is custom manufactured for each patient. Stereolithography, a rapid prototyping technology with a newer outcome in dentistry, allows the fabrication of surgical guides from 3D computer-generated models for precise placement of the implants. The surgical templates fabricated by this technology are pre-programmed with Individual depth, angulations, mesio-distal, and labio-lingual positioning of the implant to be placed. 9 Fabrication of stereolithographic templates requires the patient's computed tomography (CT) image. In CT, multiplanar reformatting allows one to reformat a volumetric dataset in sagittal, axial, and coronal cuts and also helps build multiple cross-sectional and panoramic views. Shaded surface display and volume rendering methods generate 3D reconstructions of the dental arch and its relevant structures, including nerves, making dental CT the most precise and comprehensive radiologic technique for dental implant planning. Software specially designed has been adapted to allow practitioners to virtually view the implant site and plan virtual implants' location, angle, depth, and diameter, which are superimposed on the 3D data. Following backward planning, the diagnostic wax has to be visualized through a CT scan with radiographic templates in place.

Procedures for the Fabrication of Stereolithographic Templates

1. Radiographic template
2. CT scan procedure
3. 3D computer simulation
4. Fabrication of surgical templates

A radiographic template fabricated using a radio-opaque marker is kept in the patient's mouth while the CT scan is performed. 10 During the scan, this indicates the position of the teeth and gingival tissues. During fabrication, a diagnostic wax-up is established, representing the outline of the final restoration, and is then transferred into a radiographic guide. Diagnostic casts of the dental arches are made from irreversible hydrocolloid impressions. A diagnostic wax-up of the proposed definitive restoration (in the case of an implant-supported FPD) is done.

A silicone impression of the cast with the waxed FPD is made as a mould. After retrieving the silicone impression, the waxed FPD is removed, and if the implant site is a full arch, a duplicate of a denture is made so that a radiographic stent can be made from it. A clear, chemically activated acrylic resin is poured into the mould space and cured. As an alternate, a duplicate cast is made in Type IV dental stone, and a radiographic template is made using a vacuum-formed matrix or barium sulfate as the radio-opaque marker. Access holes are made according to information obtained from the cast model, as in the case of a conventional radiographic guide. If the patient is a new denture wearer, a complete denture wax-up is done to establish denture teeth setup with phonetics, esthetics, and the proper vertical dimension of occlusion. Fabricating an ideal denture is necessary to avoid varied dimensions, which are a primary controlling factor in minimizing deviated angulations.

The radiographic template, thus fabricated, acts as a replica of the desired prosthetic result and is usually supported with different radiopaque markers such as gutta percha balls, sleeves, disks, tubes, radiopaque varnishes, lead strips or foil. Some authors prefer metal pins for better accuracy. In order to stabilize the template, the patient can be instructed to use denture adhesive during the scanning procedure. Six to eight radiopaque markers are placed in the guide if it is a completely edentulous condition. A bite index is created to ensure the correct positioning of the radiographic guide in the patient's mouth during scanning.

Understanding the underlying bony architecture and anatomic structures is a prerequisite for appropriate implant planning. In general, the quality of CT data depends on the slice thickness and the influence of possible artefacts. The thinner the slice thickness and the smaller the voxel size, the higher the resolution and accuracy of measurements of delineated structures. Movement and metallic artefacts in some dental restorations may lead to geometric distortion and an invalid acquisition.

To summarize the stereolithography fabrication process:

1. A CT scan procedure is performed with a radiographic template fabricated using radio-opaque markers in

2. Data obtained from a CT scan procedure is either sent to the master site of a specific software company, or the dentist can use the software to customize the treatment by viewing the virtual 3D model from various angles.
3. The final proposed treatment plan is sent to SLA, which scans the image and fabricates the template

Double Scan Protocol

Some authors have developed a double-scan technique for the artefact-free, high-resolution digitization of the radiographic guide. In this technique, the first scan is of the patient wearing the radiographic guide. The second scan is a scan of only the radiographic guide. Based on the spherical markers visible in both scans, the scans are superimposed onto each other, resulting in a 3D bone model of the patient and a 3D model of the radiographic guide. 12 The combination of a 3D bone model, including the 3D radiological dataset and the 3D radiographic guide model, enables the clinician to place implant locations according to anatomical, functional, and aesthetic needs and demands. In order to achieve this, the clinician virtually positions the implants with the optimal length and diameter. Any 3D location and implant type, size, or shape modifications can be done in the 3D setting or the reslice viewer. After finalizing the planning, the corresponding surgical template is designed. The surgical template thus fabricated contains all the necessary planning information and is customized according to the planned implants' location, type, and size.

Making a Computer-Aided Template

CAD-CAM is a rapid prototyping technique wherein, after the generation of a 3D treatment plan, software slices from the file are sent to a machine that fabricates the part slice by slice.

Two main methods of rapid prototyping are

1. Additive: widely used
2. Subtractive: less effective

Stereolithographic apparatus consists of a vat that contains a liquid photopolymerized resin. A laser mounted on a vat moves in sequential cross-sectional increments of 1 mm to produce a template according to slice intervals. The polymerization process of photopolymerized resin occurs in layers. Once the surface layer of the resin on laser contact gets polymerized, a mechanical table immediately below the surface layer moves down 1 mm, carrying with it the previously polymerized resin layer. The laser now polymerizes the next layer over the previously polymerized layer of the model. In stereolithography Apparatus (SLA), only 80% of the total polymerization is completed in the vat, whereas the remaining 20% can be completed in a conventional ultraviolet light curing unit. The surgical template is provided with surgical-grade stainless steel tubes with sleeves 5 mm in height, 0.2 mm wider than the osteotomy, and a drill limiting angulation deviation to 5°. The buccal window is made so that it enhances retention during surgery. Usually, three 2-mm holes are placed into the buccal surface of each side of the denture.

Advantages:

- More precise placement of implants
- Preservation of the integrity of anatomic structures
- High geometrical accuracy of 0.1 mm.
- Shorter treatment and surgery times
- Less invasive, flapless surgery, and therefore less chance of swelling
- The less post-operative strain on the dentist and patient
- Transparency of the material, which allows seeing through the model

Disadvantages:

- Lack of visibility and tactile control during surgical procedures
- Insufficient mouth opening jeopardizes the surgical procedure.
- Risk of damage to vital anatomical structures [3]

References

[1] Laederach V, Mukaddam K, Payer M, Filippi A, Kühl S. Deviations of different systems for guided implant surgery. *Clin Oral Implants Res.* 2017;28(9):1147-1151.

[2] Kattadiyil MT, Parciak E, Puri S, Scherer MD. CAD/CAM guided surgery in implant dentistry: a brief review. *Alpha Omegan.* 2014 Spring;107(1):26-31.
[3] Rohit Shah. Guided implant surgery. *Int Educ Res J.* 2017;3(11).

Chapter 11

Surgical Application of Templates

The Compu-Guide Template System allows the whole implant team—restorative doctor, implant surgeon, and dental laboratory technicians—to diagnose, plan treatment, and perform surgical and prosthetic procedures. The clinical applications described below include the Basic, Advanced, and Compu-Temp templates. Of course, where conditions warrant, the Compu-Tack template may be employed if not enough teeth are present to hold the surgical template securely during the surgery.

According to Klein, the Basic template is fabricated with drill sleeves in position to guide the initial 2 mm osteotomies to their proper locations, angles, and depths. A drilling report with the template contains the appropriate drilling measurement from the top of the drill guide sleeve for each implant site. Klein adds, "Drill depth measurement is calculated by adding the osteotomy depth, soft-tissue depth, the surgical template thickness, and the drill guide sleeve height." A drilling system is available to coordinate these drilling measurements. A doctor who wishes to control the 2 mm osteotomy location, angle, and depth would use the Basic template. At the time of surgery, visualization of the bone or anatomical structure is not necessary because the CT scan has already accomplished it. Therefore, only minimal tissue reflection is required—unless greater bone access is required to perform a bone graft or a soft-tissue procedure. After soft-tissue reflection, the surgical template is seated. The 2 mm osteotomy is created, and the template is removed. The surgery is completed conventionally. If the doctor desires, the 2 mm drill guide sleeves may be removed from a template by twisting the sleeve with a needle holder or needle-nose pliers. A 3 mm hole in the acrylic is left, which can be used to check guide pins or to check on enlarged osteotomies. "However," Klein cautions, "drilling should not be performed through this hole due to the potential for acrylic shavings to fall into the surgical wound."

The Advanced Template. The Advanced template differs from the Basic template in that the former is fabricated with a "master cylinder" inserted in the template at each of the implant locations. Klein explains, "These master cylinders accept a series of sequentially sized drill guide sleeves for each drill used during implant surgery." The Advanced template also includes a drill guide sleeve sized for the diameter of the Implant, enabling the entire drilling sequence to be performed through the template, including tapping of the implant site and placement of the Implant through the template (Figure16). An Advanced template kit contains all the drill guide sleeves, wrenches, and implant insertion tools.

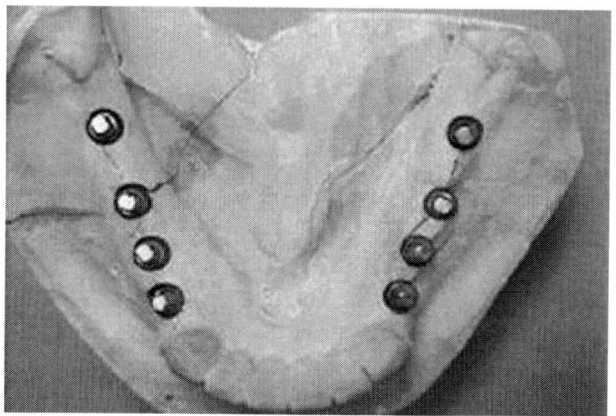

Figure 16. The Compu-Cast is a master cast of predetermined computer-milled implant positions.

The Compu-Temp Template. The Compu-Temp appliance is made with tooth-coloured teeth, as selected by the doctor, and can be made as either a Basic or advanced template. After the CT scan, this appliance is converted into the Compu-Temp surgical template, and the teeth are left to contour during this conversion fully. After the template is used for implant placement, it converts into provisional restoration. The drill guide sleeves (Basic template) or the master cylinders (Advanced template) are removed, leaving a 3 mm hole (Basic template) or a 6 mm hole (Advanced template) exactly where the implant abutment will be placed. Klein adds, "The template can be relined over the abutment and a portion of the template trimmed off, completing the provisional restoration" [1].

The fabrication of the surgical guide templates is then based on one of the following design concepts:

1. Nonlimiting design
2. Partially limiting design
3. Completely limiting design

These design concepts are classified based on the amount of surgical restriction offered by the surgical guide templates.

Nonlimiting Design

Nonlimiting designs only indicate to the surgeon where the proposed prosthesis is in relation to the selected implant site. This design indicates the ideal location of the implants without any emphasis on the angulation of the drill, thus allowing too much flexibility in the final positioning of the implant. Blustein et al. and Engelman et al. described a technique in which a guide pinhole was drilled through a clear, vacuum-formed matrix. This hole indicated the optimal position of the dental implant. However, the angulation was determined by the use of adjacent and opposing teeth. Almog et al. described the circumference lead strip guide, in which a lead strip was attached to the external surfaces of the diagnostic waxing. This was used to outline the tooth's position over the implant site. It has been observed that using these guides may result in unacceptable placement of the access hole and/or unacceptable implant angulation. Hence, these templates can serve as imaging indicators during the surgical implant placement phase. In such designs, the first drill used for the osteotomy is directed using the surgical guide, and the remainder of the osteotomy and implant placement is then finished freehand by the surgeon.

Techniques based on this design concept involve the fabrication of a radiographic template, which is then converted into a surgical guide template following radiographic evaluation. Various authors have proposed different techniques involving modifications in the following stages of fabrication: material used for the fabrication of the surgical template, radiographic marker used, type of imaging system used, and the conversion process involved in converting the radiographic template into a surgical template. Nonetheless, all the techniques mentioned above failed to restrict the angulation of the surgical drills completely.

Completely Limiting Design

A completely limiting design restricts all of the instruments used for the osteotomy in the buccolingual and mesiodistal planes. In addition, adding drill stops limits the depth of the preparation and, consequently, the positioning of the implant's prosthetic table. As the surgical guides become more restrictive, less decision-making and subsequent surgical execution are done intra-operatively. This includes two popular designs: cast-based guided surgical guides and computer-assisted design and manufacturing (CAD/CAM)-based surgical guides.

References

[1] Klein M. Implant surgery using customized surgical templates: the Compu-Guide Surgical Template System. Interview. *Dent Implantol Update.* 2002 Jun;13(6): 41-6.

Chapter 12

Advantages and Disadvantages of Templates

Benjamin notes that the surgical guide is not a panacea or intended to be used in all cases. However, in those cases where three or more implants are needed, and uncertainty exists about the bony morphology and quality of the bone, multi-planar diagnostic imaging and the surgical guide become invaluable. The fully edentulous jawbone is one of the most challenging cases confronting the implant surgeon. As bony irregularities occur and the resorption of alveolar bone progresses, internal anatomical structures become more prominent. Benjamin believes that, in such cases, "The use of multi-planar diagnostic imaging and SLA [stereolithographic] modelling for fully edentulous cases will provide accurate planning and improved postoperative results, decreased risks and shortened treatment time." Using the surgical guide as a reference during surgery, the clinician is afforded previously unavailable solutions.

As the demands of clinical practice become more challenging, applying such noninvasive diagnostic tools and technological advances in surgical technique becomes more imperative. Suppose the clinician desires a surgical guide for a single missing tooth. In that case, the minimum distance between the two neighbouring teeth (at the height of closest contact) is at least 9.2 mm, and no metal artefacts are allowed in the implant region. The minimum distance between a tooth and the centre of a planned implant is 3 mm. The advantages of the surgical guide come with a price, however, since the input data for all CADCAM diagnostic imaging is retrieved from CT technology. Benjamin explains, "Positioning and angulation of the individual jawbone become critical when metal restorations are present." Benjamin notes that pure titanium is the only metal that does not produce a flash artefact or scatter when the X-ray beam passes through it; the metal artefacts of partially edentulous jawbones, which cannot be alleviated by positioning or angulation, can cause discrepancies in the slice data, preventing the construction of a reliable surgical guide.

Benjamin suggests that the clinician, particularly the specialist, who wishes to use multi-planar diagnostic imaging and the surgical guide should contact Columbia Scientific Inc., a Materialize Company. Benjamin explains, "Columbia Scientific is the developer and distributor of the diagnostic software [Simplant] and provides CT scan protocols as well as instructions for obtaining surgical guides as a result of a practitioner's diagnostic implant plan." Of course, several software makers produce similar products. Surgical guides are often used for dental implants. However, they can also be used for more complicated surgeries, such as fixing facial bone deformities, where they have a good track record of improving both function and appearance. Finally, Benjamin notes that the evolution of multiple uses of dental implant templates (including preoperative radiography components, surgical guides, and fixed implant-supported prostheses) has led to a comprehensive implant system, helping both the patient and the clinician better manage the cost, treatment, and outcomes of implant surgery [1].

References

[1] Dunn DB. Guided implant surgery -the new "standard of care?". Australasian Dental Practice. 2009 January/February 2009.

Chapter 13

Protocols for Guided Implant Surgery

With the traditional placement of implants, restorations are made after the placement of the implants from maxillary and mandibular arch impressions, a bite registration, and diagnostic casts poured and mounted on an articulator. In guided surgery, the first step is to plan the restoration. Guided surgery may permit the placement of a restoration concomitant with the insertion of the implants by developing the restorative plan in concert with the surgical plan. A digital or analogue diagnostic tooth arrangement is created to indicate the dental anatomy and teeth positions to be replaced. A scanning prosthesis is placed in the patient's mouth, and a CT or CBCT scan is taken with the patient wearing the prosthesis. The scan is then imported into a dental software program, allowing the clinician to "virtually" place the implants into their ideal positions concerning the restoration and underlying anatomy. The digital plan is then uploaded via the Internet for guide fabrication, permitting a laboratory to fabricate the surgical guide using CADCAM technology. The surgical guide is worn by the patient during surgery and used to place the implants in the same positions, depths, and angulations as they were placed "virtually" in the planning software. To perform guided surgery, the clinician needs:

Access to a Cone-Beam CT Scanner

These CT scan machines are similar to those used to aid surgeons in joint replacement procedures but utilize much less radiation.

Implant Planning Software

Cone beam CT scanners produce images in Digital Imaging and Communications in Medicine (DICOM) format. Implant planning software reads DICOM files and reconstructs them in 2-D or 3-D images. These software packages provide various tools for implant planning, allowing the user to refer to the anatomic structure of the patient and plan a safe surgery. A wide array of implant planning software applications exist, encompassing over a dozen options such as Anatomage, NobelGuide/Nobel Clinician, Cybermed, and SimPlant.

A Surgical Template

The surgical template is a laboratory-fabricated device that references surgical planning information. Generally, it is the shape of an orthodontic splint worn by the patient during surgery. Small sleeves are inserted into the surgical template to guide the drilling. Three types of computer-generated surgical guides are available: tooth-supported, mucosa-supported, and bone-supported guides.

Guided Implant Surgery Drill Kit

A special drill kit is necessary to use a surgical template for guided surgery. This kit may include a tissue punch, a drill sleeve, and drills of various lengths and diameters that are compatible with specific guides and implant manufacturers. [1]

References

[1] Richard H. Yamada DVG. *Guided Implant Surgery*. "A Periodontal Practice Committed to Excellence." 2013.

Chapter 14

Guided Implant Surgery

Prosthetically driven implant surgery has been a fundamental interest to the dental profession. Correct implant positioning has apparent advantages, such as favourable esthetic and prosthetic outcomes, long-term stability of peri-implant hard and soft tissues due to simple oral hygiene, and the potential to ensure optimal occlusion and implant loading. Moreover, correct implant positioning enables the final prostheses to be optimally designed. It makes it possible to devise and fabricate retrievable screw-retained supra structures, thereby avoiding non-retrievable cemented restorations. Consequently, all of these factors may contribute to the long-term success of dental implants. Furthermore, various requirements, such as the desired inter-implant distance, tooth-to-implant distance, implant depth, and other aspects, have made virtual implant planning a vital tool for optimal treatment success.

In 1988, Columbia Scientific, Inc. (Glen Burnie, MD, USA) introduced three-dimensional dental software that converted computerized tomography axial slices into reformatted cross-sectional images of the alveolar ridges for diagnosis and evaluation. Consequently, in 1991, a combination software, ImageMaster-101, was introduced, which provided the additional feature of placing graphic images of dental implants on the cross-sectional images. The first version of SimPlant, produced by Columbia Scientific in 1993, allowed the placement of virtual implants of exact dimensions on cross-sectional, axial, and panoramic views of computerized tomography images. Simplant 6.0 (Columbia Scientific, 1999) added the creation of a three-dimensional reformatted image surface rendering to the software. In 2002, Materialise (Leuven, Belgium) purchased Columbia Scientific and introduced the technology for drilling osteotomies to an exact depth and direction through a surgical guide. Since then, several software, rapid prototyping, and implant companies have introduced software and surgical guide modalities to allow a guided surgical approach. Figure 17 shows the applicability of cone-beam computerized tomography imaging in conjunction with a virtual planning program. Generally, two types of guided implant surgery protocols—static and dynamic—are described in the literature. The static approach refers to the use of a static surgical template. This reproduces the virtual implant position directly from computerized tomographic data to a surgical guide, which does not allow intra-operative modification of the implant position. With static systems, a specially designed drilling machine usually transfers the planned implant location to the surgical template.

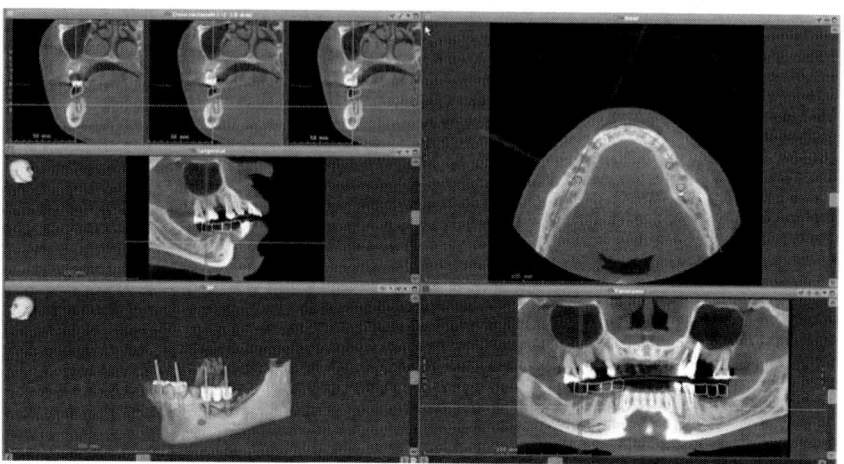

Figure 17. Virtual implant planning.

Another option called the stereolithographic method, uses specifically designed software to virtually design the surgical stent and then fabricate it using the polymerization of an ultraviolet-sensitive liquid resin. The first dynamic-guided surgery systems were introduced to implant dentistry at the beginning of the year 2000. The dynamic approach, also called navigation, refers to using a surgical navigation system to directly reproduce the virtual implant position from computerized tomographic data and allow intra-operative changes of the implant position. These systems are based on motion-tracking technology that allows real-time tracking of the dental drill and the patient throughout the entire surgery.

The introduction of cone-beam computerized tomography scanning, in combination with three-dimensional imaging tools, has led to a breakthrough in virtual implant treatment planning. Conebeam computerized tomography scanners use lower radiation doses than conventional computerized tomography scanners. Additionally, cone-beam computerized tomography scanners are much smaller and less expensive than conventional computerized tomography scanning machines, allowing the private practitioner to buy and install a conebeam computerized tomography machine in his clinical setting. Combined with implant planning software, the use of cone-beam computerized tomography data has made it possible to virtually plan the ideal implant position while considering the surrounding vital anatomic structures and future prosthetic requirements. Consequently, this process ultimately results in transferring the planned virtual implant position from the computer to the patient. In addition, intraoral scanning devices have recently started to contribute considerably to these novel treatment modalities with respect to treatment planning. By superimposing images of recognizable structures (e.g., teeth) obtained from cone-beam computerized tomography and intra-oral scanning, a more realistic digital view of a patient's dental hard and soft tissues is created. A digital setup can also be added to this data set to assist dental professionals in planning future prosthetic restoration. Nevertheless, while technology continuously improves, some significant issues must be considered when implementing these techniques to treat patients. [1]

Surgical Procedure in Brief

- *Prepare the surgical template (Figure 18).*
    - Remove any unnecessary ridges using a bur.
    - Disinfect the surgical template.
- *Secure the surgical template in place (Figure 19).*
    - Secure the surgical template into place using the bite index.
    - Drill with the anchor drill
      Insert the anchor pin in place.
- *Remove the soft tissue (Figure 20)*
    - Use the tissue punch to punch out the soft tissue.
    - Remove the anchor pin and surgical template from the patient's oral cavity.
    - Remove the soft tissue from the patient's oral cavity.
    - Place the surgical template and anchor pin back into the patient's oral cavity.
- *Drilling (Figure 21)*
    - Begin drilling with the 2.0mm drill and 2.0mm drill guide placed into the sleeve.
    - Switch to the 3.0mm drill guide and 3.0mm drill and continue drilling.

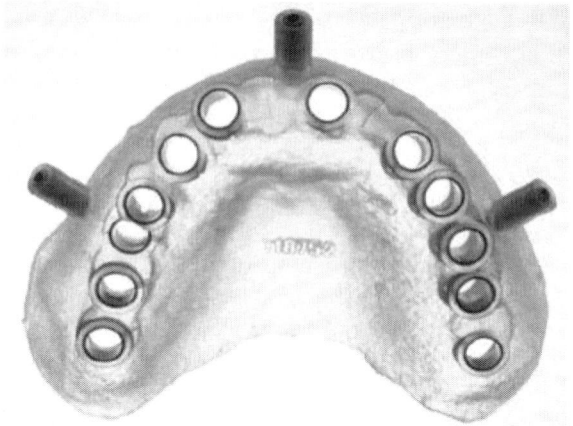

Figure 18. Prepare the surgical template.

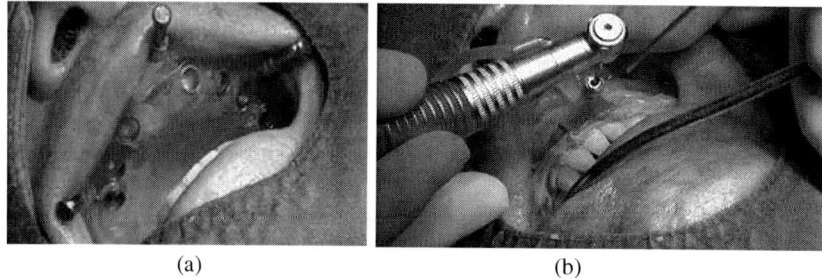

(a) (b)

Figure 19. (a),(b) Secure the surgical template in place.

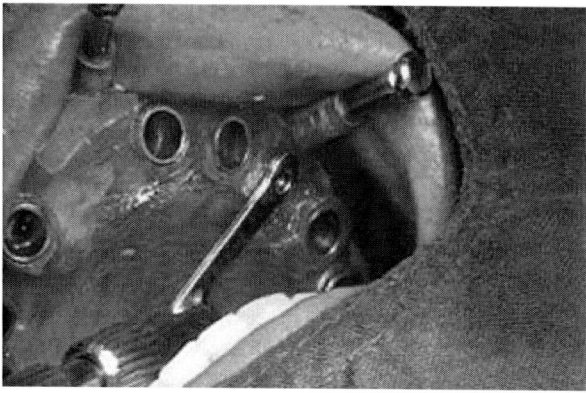

Figure 20. Remove the soft tissue.

Guided Implant Surgery

- *Implant Fixture Installation (Figure 22)*
  - Place the implant fixture onto a guided surgery mount.
  - Place the implant into the patient's oral cavity.
  - Remove the anchor pin and surgical template after all the implant fixtures are installed.
- *Placement of provisional restoration (Figure 23)*
  - Following the implant fixture installation, a provisional crown is placed over it.

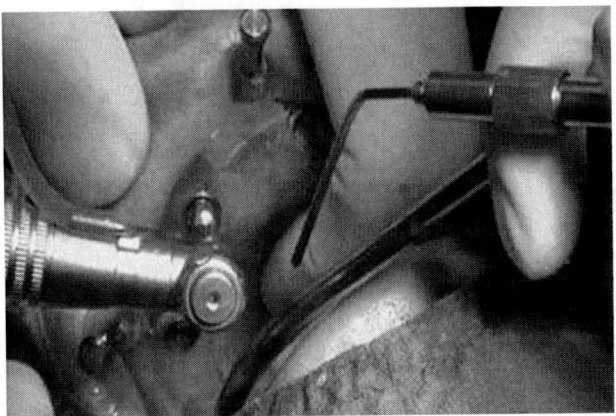

Figure 21. Drilling.

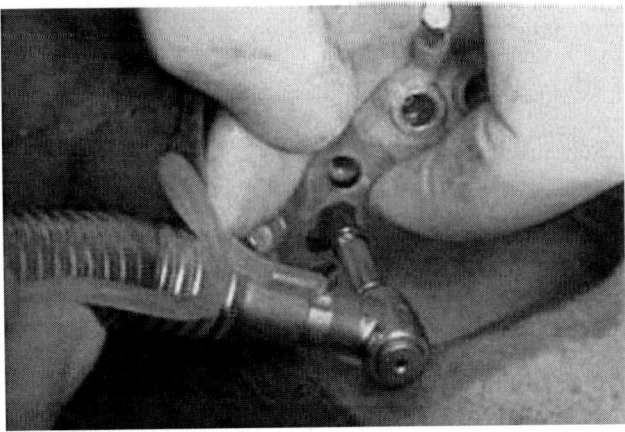

Figure 22. Implant Fixture Installation.

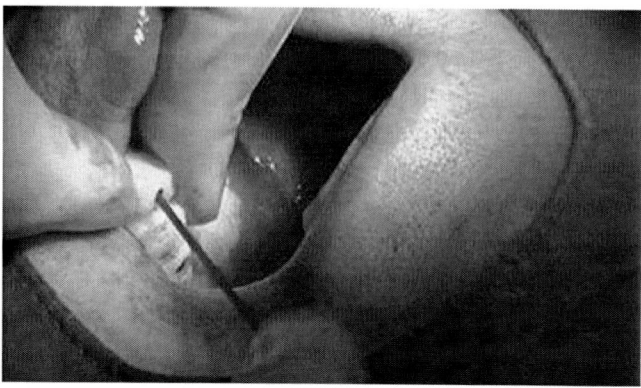

Figure 23. Placing provisional restoration.

Guided Implant Placement

It can be broadly of two types.

- The CT-based image navigation system
- CT-based surgical guide navigation system
- Both static and optical dynamic navigation systems are available for guided implant surgery.

The dynamic systems are based upon three-dimensional data, with the osteotomy drill displayed "live" at the time of surgery by infra-red optical correlation of the patient's jaw with the drill by the software and displayed on a computer screen in the surgical setting [2].

References

[1] Albiero AM, Benato R, Momic S, Degidi M. Implementation of computer-guided implant planning using digital scanning technology for restorations supported by conical abutments: A dental technique. *J Prosthet Dent.* 2018;119(5):720-726.

[2] *Navigation surgery*. Dental council of north america.

Chapter 15

CT Based Guided Implant Surgery

These systems provide sensors and software to transfer the pre-surgical plan to the patient, indicating when the dentist placing the implants has physically deviated from the predetermined drilling parameters. They also provide automated monitoring of the surgical process. The procedure is limited by the physical navigation control of the dentist placing the implants and the fact that the sensing device is sensitive to the line of sight.

The sequence of steps in image-guided surgery:

- Data acquisition
- Identification
- Registration
- Navigation

Data Acquisitions

CT and CBCT scans are widely used for 3D patient imaging. The patient is scanned for image data acquisition with radiopaque markers. Artificial or natural radiographic markers are used. For example, stents with markers intentionally placed pins or screws in the jaw or natural markers such as teeth or bony landmarks. If artificial markers are placed in a stent, the patient must have it in place when scanned.

Identification

Jaws are interpreted by software as anatomical geometric elements. Several devices have been used to capture patient anatomy for registration with scanned data, including a touch pointer and an ultrasound probe. The touch pointer allows the operator to touch specific anatomic points while the tracking device sees the instrument and records each point of reference. This device is relatively accurate, but if the clinician is not careful, there may be false mapping. The ultrasonic probe has a lower accuracy but has the advantage of being able to capture continuous data on bone morphology through the mucosa.

Registration

Initially, information regarding the patient's position about the navigation system has to be relayed. This procedure is called registration. It is performed according to various principles. Traditionally, the head of the anaesthetized patient is fixed in the holding device, which in turn is screwed onto the operating field.

Before the first incision, the properly fixed skin markers on the patient are touched with the probe tip of the navigation instrument with the CT or MRI. Simultaneously, it shows the probe tip position as a crosshair in the original layers and two vertically computed levels on the screen. The 3D reconstruction of the CT data is shown in the fourth screen window, which displays both the positions and the orientation of the whole probe and a projected virtual extension of the probe axis.

Navigation

The intraoperative instrument navigation system aims to support the surgeon through the localization of anatomical regions and guide the use of surgical instruments.

Instrument navigation can be done through

- Mechanical tracking systems
- Magnetic tracking systems
- Optical tracking systems
- Ultrasound-based systems

Chapter 16

CAD Cam Based Guided Implant Surgery

Technique

Presurgical procedure:

1. Prepare mounted diagnostic casts with fully extended vestibular borders of the edentulous space. On those casts, complete a diagnostic waxing or use acrylic resin artificial teeth to identify the ideal tooth positions for replacing missing teeth.
2. Duplicate the diagnostic tooth arrangement in acrylic resin (Jet Tooth Shade; Lang Dental Mfg. Co., Wheeling, Ill). On the cast, block out the buccal and lingual undercuts of the teeth with wax (Truwax; Dentsply International, York, Pa.) and coat the existing teeth with a separator (Rubber Sep; George Taub Products and Fusion, Jersey City, NJ). Add 3 to 4 mm of acrylic resin to the occlusal surface of the existing teeth, extending the acrylic resin into the lingual vestibule of the mandibular arch or the palate in the maxilla. Do not cover the occlusal surface of the acrylic resin teeth; cover only the buccal and lingual surfaces to attach the teeth to the template (Figure 24).
3. Make three verification windows (occlusal openings in the radiographic template to view the occlusal surface of the teeth through the template, confirming the seating of the radiographic and surgical templates) with an acrylic bur (Laboratory Carbide Cutter H251FSQ; Brasseler USA, Savannah, Ga.) around the arch of the
4. Make six to eight 1.5- to 2.0-mm-diameter holes in the vestibular borders of the radiographic template.

Place the holes from the cervical plane to the gingival plane. Make the holes in the approximate positions of the central incisors, canines, premolars, and molars, and fill them with gutta-percha (Gutta-percha; The Hygenic Corp., Akron, Ohio).

1. Make an interocclusal record with a rigid vinyl polysiloxane (Access Blue: Centrix Dental, Shelton, Conn.) for the patient to hold the radiographic template in position during the CT scan and prevent movement. Make the record intraorally or on the mounted cast at the initial contact of the radiographic template.
2. Prescribe a CT scan of the arch with the edentulous space using a double scan. Make the first scan of the patient with the radiographic template in place. Make the second scan of the radiographic template only.
3. Download the CT data onto the computer. Convert the CT data in the surgical software (Procera Software CT scan file converter application; Nobel Biocare), superimposing the two sets of scans (one of the osseous tissues and the other of the radiographic template) to show the planned position of the teeth in relation to the Using the 3-D implant planning software (Procera Planning Software; Nobel Biocare), evaluate the osseous tissues in relation to the position of the teeth through the merging of independent data. From this information, evaluate and plan the positions and sizes of the dental implants.
4. After the plan is complete, transfer the data to a milling centre (Procera; Nobel Biocare) to fabricate the stereolithography surgical template via a CAD/CAM procedure, with the implant positioning sleeves (Guided Sleeves; Nobel Biocare) cemented in the surgical.
5. Evaluate and adjust the surgical template to ensure proper seating on the cast, and Adjust the acrylic resin rings around each of the guide sleeves so that they do not interfere with the seating of the template.
6. Place the adjusted surgical template onto the cast on which the radiographic template was fabricated. Cut a space in the cast for implant analogues with a carbide bur (Laboratory Carbide Cutter H79FSQ; Brasseler USA). Position the implant analogues in the template with transfer copings (Guided Cylinder with Pin Unigrip; Nobel Biocare) to provide the exact positions of the implants in the x-, y-, and z-axes (this transfer does not locate any orientation of the implant's external hex or lobes of an internally connected implant). Place a soft tissue replica (Gi-Mask; Coltene/Whaledent, Cuyahoga Falls, Ohio) into the template and around the implant.
7. Add ADA type II dental stone (Denstone; Heraeus Kulzer, South Bend, Ind.) to the cast and implant analogues to connect the analogues to the cast.

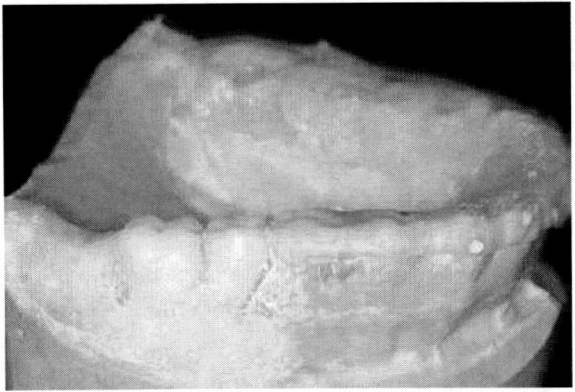

Figure 24. Radiographic template with buccal and lingual vestibular border extensions.

8. Fabricate a provisional or definitive restoration on the cast if an immediate load procedure is planned. For the patient presented, a splinted acrylic resin (Jet Tooth Shade Acrylic Resin; Lang Dental Mfg Co.) provisional restoration was fabricated using nonengaging copings (Snappy Abutment temporary copings; Nobel Biocare). Place the selected abutments (Snappy Abutments; Nobel Biocare) onto the working cast. Place the nonengaging copings on the abutments. Using a vacuform matrix (0.020", clear temporary splint material; Buffalo Dental, Syosset, NY) made of the original diagnostic waxing, place acrylic resin into the vacuum-formed matrix, filling the void from the matrix to the provisional

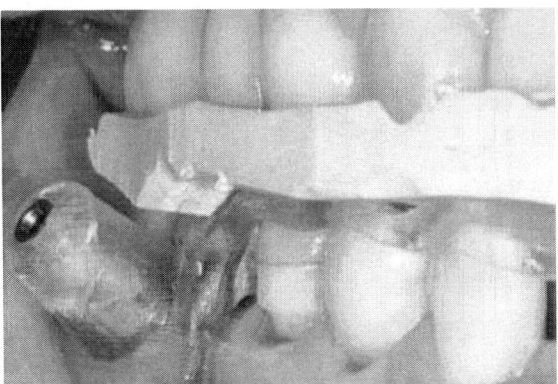

Figure 25. Surgical templates in place.

9. Make an interocclusal record with a rigid vinyl polysiloxane (Access Blue; Centrix Dental) between the surgical template and the opposing arch on the patient or the mounted cast (Figure 25).

Surgical Procedure

1. After the local anaesthetic is given, place the surgical template intraorally. Confirm the seating of the template through the verification windows. Have the patient occlude into the interocclusal record made in the laboratory between the surgical template and the opposing arch.
2. Place the friction-fitted horizontal stabilization pins (NobelGuide Anchor Pins; Nobel Biocare) to hold the surgical template with a 1.5-mm twist drill to the planned. Once seated, have the patient open to expose the surgical sites of the guide.
3. Prepare each implant site first using a start drill (NobelGuide Start Drill; Nobel Biocare), a soft tissue punch and a counter-sink drill. Using the surgical template, guide the start drill in the correct x-, y-, and z-axes. Next, place a 2-mm drill guide into the surgical template. Use the 2-mm drill through the guide to control the x- and y-axes to the planned implant depth. Use the appropriate-sized drills to expand the osteotomy site for the planned implant diameter and length. Complete the osteotomy site and place the implant with an implant mount (NobelGuide Surgical Implant Mount; Nobel Biocare) to control the implant position's x-axis, y-axis, and z-axis, replicating the planned position in the surgical planning software.
4. After placing the implants, attach the abutments (Snappy Abutments) and cement the restoration (Figure 26). Use definitive cement (Ketac-Cem Aplicap; 3M ESPE, St. Paul, Minn.) to prevent loosening of the restoration. Line the restoration with cement. Do not overfill the restoration with cement. Ensure all excess cement is removed around the abutment and implant. Adjust the provisional restoration out of occlusion to prevent implant overload and micromovements.
5. Evaluate the patient postoperatively for lateral contacts and healing. Examine the patient for lateral interferences and healing at 1-, 2-, and 4-week intervals and three months following. After implant integration is determined, fabricate the definitive restorations [1].

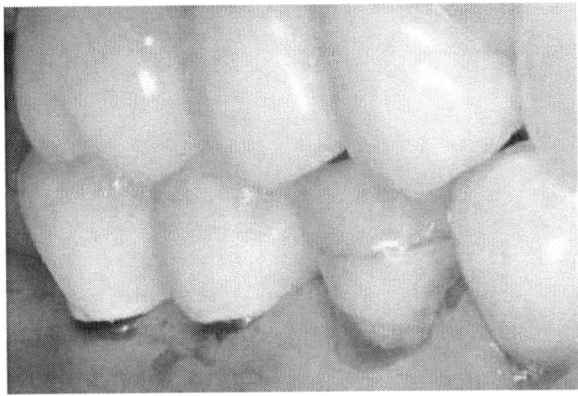

Figure 26. Splinted provisional restoration, seated on abutments.

References

[1] Dunn DB. Guided implant surgery -the new "standard of care?". Australasian Dental Practice. 2009 January/February 2009.

Chapter 17

Cast Based Guided Implant Surgery

A fully restrictive surgical guide allows controlled execution of a preoperatively planned osteotomy and subsequent implant placement. There are two fabrication modes. One is a digital path, where these guides can be fabricated based on data from a cone-beam CT source. Alternatively, 3-D data can be derived from a dental cast and periapical radiographs. The 3D Click Guide is a cast-based, fully restrictive surgical guide that can be generated in the dental office.

An overextended impression is taken to capture the maximum of the edentulous ridge. Either alginate or vinyl polysiloxane can be used. A stock tray is filled with stiff VPS putty (Examix, GC America Inc., Alsip, Ill.) and covered with a thin sheet of food foil (Saran Wrap, SC Johnson, Racine, Wis.). Once placed in the mouth, finger pressure pushes the putty against the lingual and buccal soft tissues. This will result in a tight adaptation of the soft tissue against the bone. Upon setting, a small portion of new putty is mixed and added to the buccal and lingual areas of the impression at the treatment area. This is covered with food foil and placed back in the mouth. The additional force will push down the soft tissue and actively overextend the impression. Remove the tray from the mouth and remove the foil. This pre impression is now filled with injection-grade VPS material and repositioned. The resulting impression has captured a much larger area of the crest than we are commonly used to in dentistry. Alternatively, a stock tray is extended by locally applying orthodontic rope wax (Wax square ropes, Patterson Dental Supply, St. Paul, Minn.) at the site of interest, in the mandible, both lingual and buccal, and in the maxilla, just buccal. Alginate is mixed to a stiff consistency, and the tray is filled. The tray is positioned in the mouth; the soft wax will push the tissues down, exposing the alveolar ridge. A topical anaesthetic is placed on the soft tissue of the edentulous site (Figure 27). The soft tissue thickness is measured using a 27-gauge short anaesthetic needle (Fairfax Dental, Miami) with an endodontic rubber stopper; five readings are taken per implant (Figure 28).

- Deep buccal = 2 mm above the deepest point captured by impression capture.
- High buccal = 3–4 mm below crest
- Deep lingual = 2 mm above the deepest point captured by impression
- High lingual = 3–4 mm below the crest
- Crest can also be measured by X-ray.

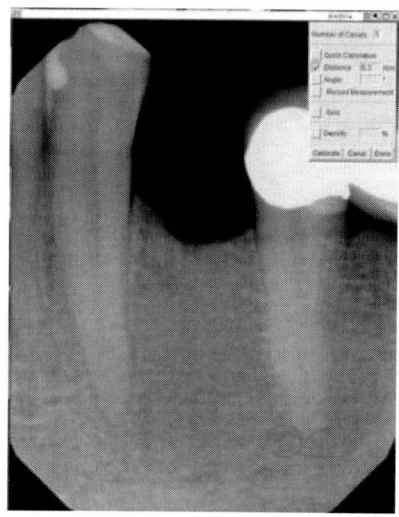

Figure 27. Preoperative radiograph, marked mental foramen and estimated length of implant.

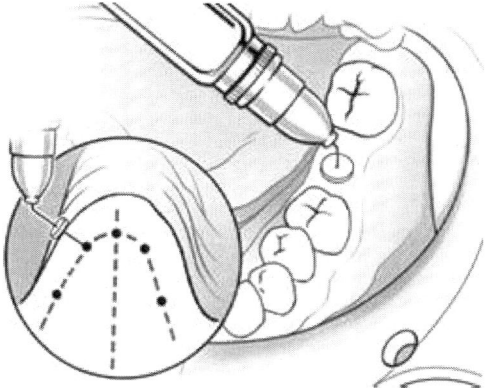

Figure 28. Topical anesthetic allows simple bone sounding with dental needle.

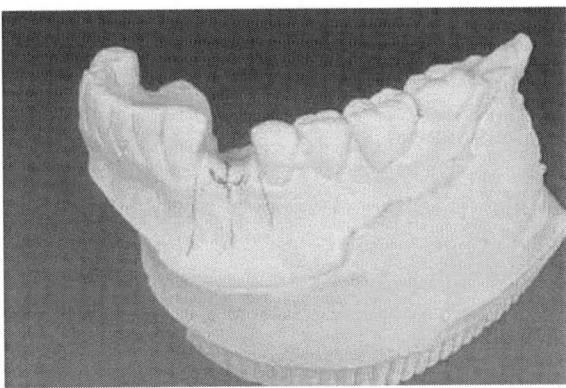

Figure 29. Stone cast from overextended impression, capturing edentulous ridge.

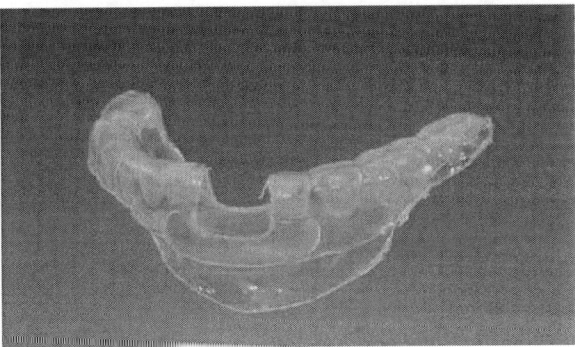

Figure 30. Dual layered vacuform carrier.

The impression is poured into an Accu-Trac Precision Die System tray (Coltene/Whaledent Inc., Cuyahoga Falls, Ohio) or DVA twin trays (Dental Ventures of America Inc., Corona, Calif.) using dental stone (Earth Stone, Tak System Inc., Wareham, Mass.) or VPS casting material (Blu-Mousse/Mach 2 Slow, Parkell Inc., Edgewood, N.Y.). Alternatively, a Pindex system can be used (Figure 29). A denture tooth or wax-up is placed. The buccal gingival outline of the desired prosthetic outcome is marked. The shoulder of the implant should generally be 2–3 mm below this line.

A dual-layer vacuform carrier is created. Using 1 mm soft-guard material and 0.75 mm bondable material, which are heated together (Essix A+ and model duplication material, Dentsply Raintree Essix, Sarasota, Fla.) (Figure 30). The cast is cut along the mesiodistal (MD) path of the proposed MD axis for the implant. The cut is based on estimating neighbouring roots and the centre of the tooth that will be replaced. A radiograph and anatomical information are used as references. The five tissue-thickness readings are transferred to the cut face of the cast, and the markings are connected parallel to the soft tissue.

The desired buccolingual (BL) implant axis is marked on the cast relative to bone volume and wax. The desired top of the implant is determined, followed by drilling one mm-diameter hole at the implant axis. The top of the implant is generally 2–3 mm below the buccal gingival outline. This placement will put the top surface of the rotation block 9 mm above the shoulder of the implant (9 + 1 = 10 mm above the drill guide). The blue buccolingual positioner (BLP) is placed in the hole and lined up with the drawn axis. Fast-setting cyanoacrylate glue secures the positioner (Instant Krazy Glue, Krazy Glue, Columbus, Ohio).) Some cast material is removed from the opposing part of the BLP. The parts of the cast are placed back into an Accu-trac tray, DVA twin trays, or a Pindexed cast. The correction slot of the buccal wing is positioned on top of the BLP. The wings of the radiographic implant replicas (RIRs) are cut or bent as needed for a passive fit. The lingual wing (white) is attached and adjusted. The complete assembly is positioned atop the BLP (Figure 31). The wings and RIRs are secured with a fast-setting poly(methyl methacrylate) (PMMA) ortho-acrylic (Orthodontic Resin, Dentsply, York, Penn.) to create an irreversible solid connection. The cross member is removed, exposing the retention rails (Figure 32). The surgical guide is placed in the mouth, and a radiograph is taken. If the radiograph is exposed perpendicular to the ridge, then the images of the two RIRs will overlap and appear as one. This indicates a diagnostically appropriate image. If the trajectory is as desired, no rotational corrections are needed; then a 0-degree rotation block (green) is selected. If a minor correction is warranted, a 3-degree yellow rotation block is selected (Figure 33). A more extensive correction is possible by selecting a 7-degree red rotation block. A small-diameter initial drill is selected depending on the manufacturer's drilling protocol. Drill with the 2.0 mm pilot drill to a short and safe depth and evaluate the length of the osteotomy. The top of the rotation block is 9 mm above the top of the implant. The drill guide is 1 mm thick, so the drill stop should be set at +10 mm for accurate depth control. For example, a 10-mm osteotomy requires the drill stop to be set at 10 + 10 = 20 mm. The final length of the implant can then be determined, and the osteotomy can be prepared to that length. Subsequent drills of larger diameter are employed to widen the osteotomy as required (Figure 34). The implant can now be placed using guidance and depth control (Figure 35) [1].

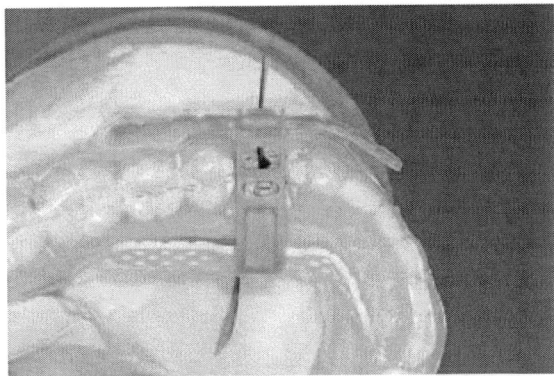

Figure 31. The buccal and lingual wings are positioned for the desired mesiodistal position, while maintaining the previously selected buccolingual position.

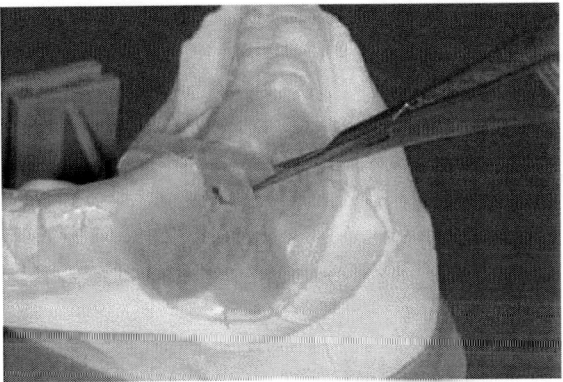

Figure 32. The wings are attached to the vacuform carrier with ortho-acrylic.

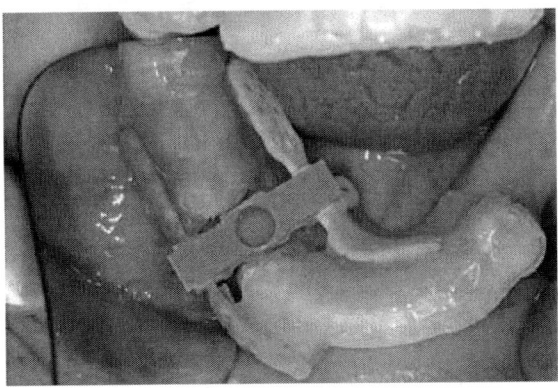

Figure 33. A yellow 3-degree rotation block is selected.

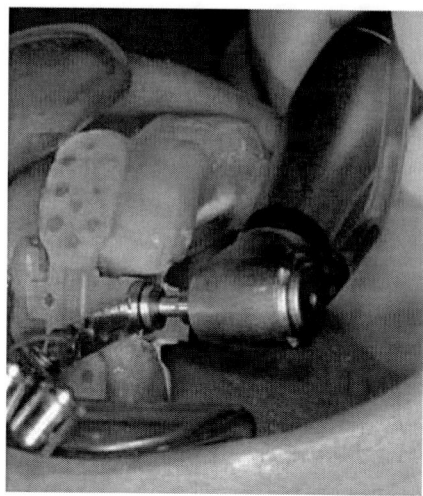

Figure 34. 3.2 mm osteotomy for an 8 mm implant.

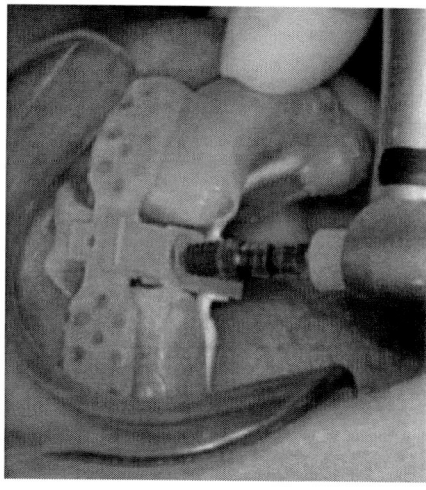

Figure 35. Implant ready for visually guided implant placement.

References

[1] Vercruyssen M, Cox C, Naert I, Jacobs R, Teughels W, Quirynen M. Accuracy and patient-centered outcome variables in guided implant surgery: a RCT comparing immediate with delayed loading. *Clin Oral Implants Res.* 2016;27(4):427-32.

Chapter 18

CBCT Guided Flapless Implant Surgery

Various flapless implant surgical techniques can be used for flapless implant surgery; these include free hand, CBCT guided, and CBCT guided and navigated flapless implant surgery. A systematic review by Voulgarakis et al. compared the outcomes of these three flapless surgical procedures, assessing implant survival rates and marginal bone loss. Twenty-three studies with a minimum of 1-year follow-up were included. The following results were reported: free-hand flapless implant surgery demonstrated 98.3–100% implant survival rates and mean marginal bone loss of between 0.09 and 1.40 mm 1-4 years after implant insertion. Flapless CBCT-guided surgery (without 3D navigation) had an implant survival rate of between 91–100% and a mean marginal bone loss of 0.89 mm after an observation period of 2–10 years, and CBCT-guided and navigated flapless surgery showed implant survival rates of between 89–100% and a mean marginal bone loss of between 0.55–2.6 mm over a follow-up period of 1–5 years. This systematic review concluded that there are several methods to facilitate implant placement via a flapless approach and that none of the methods demonstrated has advantages over the others with regard to implant survival and marginal bone loss. However, D'hase et al. suggested that free-hand flapless implant surgery can only be advocated in specific, pre-planned cases by experienced surgeons with adequate bone volume.

- Proposed factors that can lead to errors and inaccuracies in the production of CBCT surgical implant guides
- CBCT scan quality.
- File conversion and reformatting of the CBCT scan The CBCT implant planning software used
- The type of production methods used for the surgical guide, with CAM-manufactured CBCT surgical guides being more accurate than lab-constructed guides (non-CAM),
- The material used to construct the surgical guides, as there are reports of surgical guide fracturing during surgical use.

- The ability to position the surgical guide accurately at the time of surgery
- The type of support the surgical guide has (tooth, bone, mucosa or soft tissue) is determined by the type of guide, with tooth-supported guides shown to have more accurate implant positioning than bone-supported guides.
- The ability of the surgical guide to remain stable during use, with the increasing use of fixation screws, has been shown to reduce implant deviations.
- The surgeon's experience in using such guides
- Access to the surgical site or position of the edentulous area has also been reported as a source of inaccuracies leading to implant deviations. [1]

Surgical Procedures

Pre-Operative Instructions

Patients were instructed to take systemic antibiotics (amoxicillin 500mg, 3x/d, five days) and ibuprofen 600mg 1 day and 1 hour prior to surgery, respectively. After administering local anaesthetics, patients were instructed to rinse with a 0.12% chlorhexidine solution for 30 seconds. Thereupon, surgery was performed according to the treatment the patients had been assigned to. All surgeries were performed by the same experienced clinician (FY), and all implants were OsseoSpeed® EV of various dimensions (Astra Tech Implant System®, Dentsply Sirona Implants, Mölndal, Sweden).

Free-Handed Surgery

Before surgery, only images from the software planning and rough distance calculations were allowed as references. After making a crystal and sulcular incision on the neighbouring teeth, a full-thickness mucoperiosteal flap was raised on the buccal and palatal sides. Subsequent osteotomies were prepared according to the manufacturer's guidelines, considering specific anatomical landmarks visible on the pre-operative CBCT (roots of neighbouring teeth, sinus floor, undercuts). After preparation, implants were installed according to the manufacturer's guidelines. If the insertion torque failed to reach 15 Ncm, a cover screw was placed, and the flap was closed on top. If an insertion torque of >15 Ncm was achieved, a healing abutment was installed, and after careful recontouring of the palatal mucosa, soft tissues were closed around it. Non-resorbable monofilament sutures (Seralon® 5/0, Serag-Wiessner, Naila, Germany) were used at all times.

Pilot-Drill-Guided Surgery

Pilot-drill surgery was performed without flap elevation. The fit of the surgical guide was checked and adjusted if necessary. The first osteotomy was performed with the surgical guide in situ using a 1.95-mm pilot drill. A drill stop ensured that the correct depth was reached.

According to the virtual 3D plan. Subsequent osteotomies were performed freehandedly according to the manufacturer's instructions. The depth of the osteotomy was determined as follows: A pilot drill was inserted in the primary osteotomy; the corresponding depth marking on the drill was considered, and subsequent free-handed drillings were performed according to that marking. As described above, implants were installed in a one- or two-stage procedure, depending on their primary stability. A collagen sponge (Spongostan®, Ethicon Inc., Somerville, New Jersey, USA) was sutured over the implants installed with a two-stage procedure.

Fully-Guided Surgery

Fully-guided surgery was performed without flap elevation. The fit of the surgical guide was checked and adjusted if necessary. All the osteotomies were performed with the surgical guide in situ. For each separate drill, a removable corresponding drilling tube was first inserted into the guiding sleeves to allow for fluent guiding of the drill—markings on the drills related to the depth of the osteotomy. After preparation, implants were installed with the surgical guide in situ. Semi-lunar markings on the implant driver and the guide itself ensured the correct vertical placement and alignment of the internal connection of the implant. As described above, implants were installed in a one- or two-stage procedure, depending on their primary stability. A collagen sponge (Spongostan®, Ethicon Inc., Somerville, New

Jersey, USA) was sutured over the implants installed with a two-stage procedure.

Post-Operative Instructions

Cold packs were administered immediately after surgery, and patients were instructed to continue taking antibiotics and analgesics if necessary. In addition, a 0.12% chlorhexidine solution was advocated to be used twice daily for seven days. Sutures were removed after seven days.

Post-Operative CBCT

Implants were left to integrate for 12 weeks. After removing the healing abutments or uncovering the implants, and removing the cover screws in the case of a second-stage procedure, a second CBCT was taken with the same settings and FOV as mentioned before.

Prosthetic Procedures

Implants were loaded with solitary, a prior screw-retained restorations following an osseointegration period of 3 months. Restorations were cemented Only when screw-retained restorations were not possible (e.g., screw holes exiting from the buccal side). All restorations consisted of a metal-ceramic crown on a standard titanium abutment (TiDesignTM EV, Astra Tech Implant System® EV, Dentsply Sirona Implants, Mölndal, Sweden) [2].

References

[1] Fauroux MA, De Boutray M, Malthiéry E, Torres JH. New innovative method relating guided surgery to dental implant placement. *J Stomatol Oral Maxillofac Surg.* 2018;119(3):249-253.

[2] Marlière DAA, Demètrio MS, Picinini LS, Oliveira RG, Netto HDMC. Accuracy of computer-guided surgery for dental implant placement in fully edentulous patients: A systematic review. *Eur J Dent.* 2018;12(1):153-160.

Chapter 19

Image Guided Implant Surgery

Dental implants are arguably one of the most historically significant developments in dentistry. Initially, when the current screw-shaped implants embedded in bone were introduced, surgical specialists were the leading providers of this service, and a second clinician typically restored the implant. At first, there was little joint ownership of the implant, but that scenario has changed. Today, if two providers are involved, there is generally good communication between the surgeon and restorative dentist. Surgical challenges frequently involve losing tissue support (bone and soft tissue) that does not always allow implants to be placed in an ideal position for the prosthetic superstructure. In addition, as treatments have become increasingly complex, the importance of information sharing and collaboration between surgeons and restorative doctors has increased proportionately.

Digital technology dramatically aids this communication in the initial stages of treatment by allowing three-dimensional (3D) information that details the availability of bone and the ideal position of the restoration via cone beam computed tomography (CBCT) with a radiographic guide that can later be converted to a surgical guide. Recent advances in computer aided design and manufacturing (CAD/CAM) allow the fabrication of highly accurate surgical guides that facilitate precise implant positioning.

More specifically, CAD technology can be used in implant surgery by taking CBCT images and using specialized software to place implants virtually. The resulting imaging can be shared between the surgeon, restorative dentist, and laboratory (Figure 36). This is an excellent communication tool and helps reduce discrepancies between the desired and actual implant positioning. The CBCT will show the surgeon where the crown will be from the radiographic guide, the restorative doctor can see where the surgeon plans to place the implant (based on the availability of bone), and the laboratory can provide valuable input to the surgeon and restorative doctor. If the position of the implant is acceptable to all parties, the radiographic template can be converted into a manually fabricated surgical guide, or modifications can be made. It is also possible to place virtual restorations on the implant without a radiographic template. In addition, clinicians can superimpose the CBCT on the patient's 3D scans or stone models (Figure 37), with or without wax-ups.

Besides virtual treatment planning, providers can implement all-digital workflows, from scanned impressions to surgical placement through a 3D-image-guided template and, ultimately, the milling of the restoration. As expected, approaches to fabricating surgical guides have evolved over the last 15 years. At first, the guides were designed to be placed on bone, soft tissue, and later on teeth (Figure 38). This technology requires excellent accuracy to yield predictable outcomes, and this article will address this issue in detail.

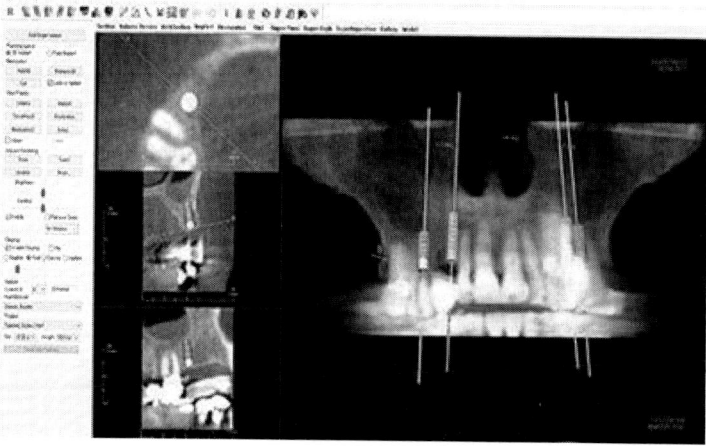

Figure 36. Available from various companies, special implant software — such as this Anatomage Invivo example — aids clinicians in virtual treatment planning.

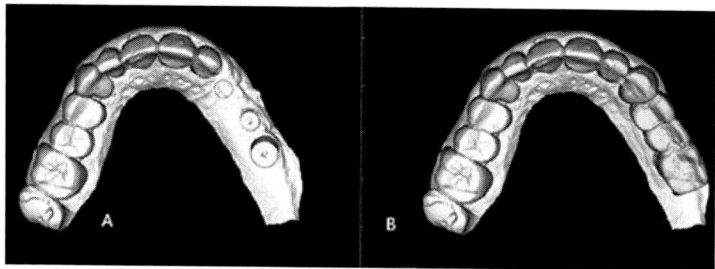

Figures 37. Stone model without wax-up (A), and with wax-up (B) scanned and superimposed on a cone beam computed tomogram virtual treatment plan for implant #11.

Placing 3D-image-guided implants entails two levels of "completeness," leading to the distinction between fully and partially guided. Assuming adequate keratinized gingiva, the fully guided approach allows flapless surgery, complete drilling with vertical control of the drills through the guide, and implant placement with a vertical stop (Figure 39). At this time, however, not all implant products allow a fully guided approach. In a partially guided technique, there may be vertical control on some of the drills, but the implant is not placed through the guide with vertical control. This typically means that it is not flapless surgery. These guides are still helpful, albeit slower and possibly not as accurate as fully guided systems, although there may be insufficient data to support that statement.

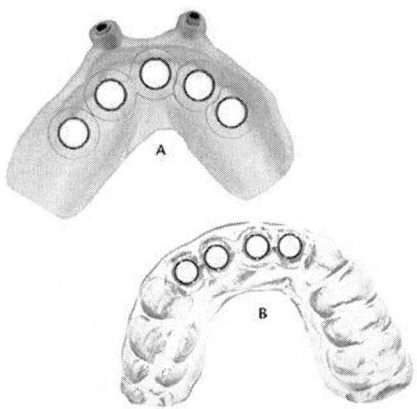

Figures 38. These images illustrate a soft tissue-borne guide with pin fixation (a), and a tooth-borne guide (b).

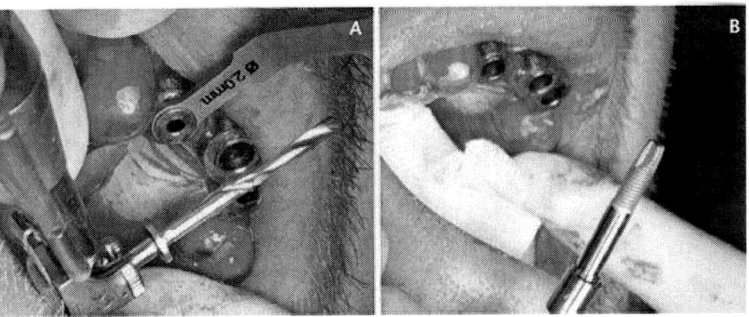

Figures 39. Three-dimensional-image-guided surgery with vertical control of drilling (A) and implant placement (B).

Surgical Accuracy

Like all developing technologies, CBCT-image-guided implant surgery has evolved through several generations of imaging and fabrication processes. The first guides were designed to be placed on the bone and fabricated using stereolithography (3D) printing technology. An early comprehensive report on this approach by van Steenberghe et al. evaluated edentulous patients receiving multiple implants with an immediate loading protocol. Conventional implant surgery almost always includes exposing the implant site with an incision and flap. However, with the additional 3D information about the architecture of the underlying bone, it has been one of the alluring aspects of guided surgery to avoid an incision and flap. This means the guide is placed and held on soft tissue, osteotomies are performed, and implants are placed with a guide based on the CBCT plan. One of the first studies of flapless image-guided surgery was by Merli et al., whose team avoided flap and bone exposure by using a computer-guided approach in the edentulous maxilla in a pilot prospective case series involving 13 patients receiving 89 implants. The researchers used Procera software and a NobelGuide approach to place the implants in atrophic, fully edentulous patients. The team noted a 94.4% implant success rate, which is similar to nonguided approaches for the atrophic edentulous maxilla. While the authors did not report data regarding accuracy, they commented that a learning curve was evident in that many of the failures occurred in the early cases.

Recent studies reported similar or slightly lower success rates with the same approach. In 2008, a paper on a flapless technique with NobelGuide was published by Komiyama et al. in this study, 29 edentulous patients received 1176 implants in an immediately loaded approach. The team noted an 89% implant success rate but a higher-than-normal incidence of surgical and technical complications. They concluded that this methodology should be considered in the exploratory phase of development. A long-term survival study by Orentlicher et al. detailed a 7-year retrospective analysis of the cumulative survival rate of implants placed using the fully guided approach. They analyzed 796 implants placed using CBCT-guided surgery in 177 patients. The cumulative survival rate was 96.9%, and they reported no reduction in survival when immediately loading the implants. Similar survival results were noted by Vasak et al. in reviewing 163 implants in 30 patients, the team reported a cumulative survival rate of 98.8%. In cases involving partially edentulous patients, though it would make sense to use the remaining teeth for placement and anchorage of the guide, achieving a good representation of the teeth in the CBCT may prove difficult. In 2008 and 2009, companies began experimenting with 3D scanning of stone models (and, later, direct intraoral scans). When superimposed in the CBCT, these scans overcame the problem of inaccurate representation of the teeth, especially when metal is present.

Fabrication and Guide Seating

It is crucial to differentiate outcomes based on the fabrication process and the guide seating method used. In 2009, Ozan et al. compared tooth-, bone-, and soft-tissue-supported guides and reported accuracy and outcomes based on seating methods. This was one of the first studies to compare the accuracy between the planned and actual position of the implant using these various approaches to seating the surgical guide. The study demonstrated the most excellent accuracy when using tooth-supported guides. The increased accuracy of guides placed on teeth was confirmed by Arisan et al. in a study of 3D-printed guides placed on teeth, bone, or soft tissue. They found tooth-borne guides significantly more accurate than either bone- or soft-tissue-supported guides. The researchers also noted that if soft-tissue-borne guides are used, accuracy could be improved by fixing the guide with screws. This has subsequently become even clearer. A recent systematic review of computer technology applications in surgical implant dentistry by Tahmaseb et al. found 14 survival and 24 accuracy studies that met the criteria for inclusion. The survival rates and accuracy reported were similar to earlier studies. Behneke et al. studied factors that affected transfer accuracy and found that flapped or flapless surgery did not significantly influence accuracy. Improved accuracy was noted, however, when the implant was placed fully guided (i.e., all drill steps and implant placement occur through the guide), as compared to freehand placement of the implant, with all drilling done guided, and when the final drill sequence was freehand and only the first drill(s) guided. These studies illustrate additional variables that are not well documented in the literature: whether the guide was used for the initial (pilot) drill or subsequent drills and if the implant was placed through the guide with a vertical stop or by freehand. Further studies are needed to understand the impact of these variables fully.

In-Office Guide Printing

The increasing quality and availability of personal 3D printers make in-office printing an attractive alternative to buying guides from laboratories (Figure 40). A downside to 3D printing technology is that, at present, these are resin-only guides. By comparison, other guides may contain

- metal sleeves that allow greater stability for drill guidance,
- all drilling is to occur through the guide, and
- the possibility of placing implants through the guide with vertical control.

In all likelihood, however, it is only a matter of time before in-office 3D printing technology catches up.

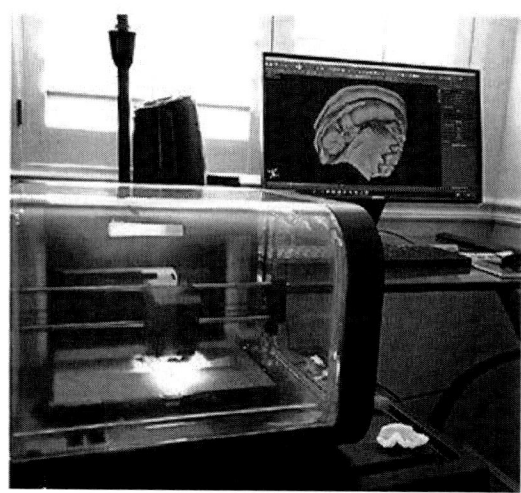

Figure 40. Advanced technology allows in-office printing of implant surgical guides.

Complications

Most studies focusing on the survival of implants placed using traditional or guided methods have not found significant differences in the ultimate complication: implant failure. The majority of these studies were retrospective in design. However, in a prospective mono-center study, researchers reviewed

26 patients receiving 114 implants with 3D imaging guides and found the 1-year survival of the implants was 88.6%; when looking at smokers and nonsmokers, the survival rates were 69.2% and 98.7%, respectively. They concluded that smoking might be considered a contraindication to guided implant surgery. In this study, some implants were placed in edentulous or partially edentulous patients, and all were placed flapless. Some implants were immediately loaded, with a higher failure rate than devices not loaded immediately. Other studies, however, have yet to report similar failure rates, neither with immediate loading nor in heavy smokers. Further research is needed to explain these variations.

Robotic Surgery

The use of navigation is an emerging approach to implant placement. Also called robotic surgery, this involves using tracking devices attached to the patient and an implanted handpiece. These two positions in space are relayed to a central processing unit and superimposed on a monitor. Their relation to the previously planned implant osteotomy is displayed, and the implant handpiece can be adjusted by following the onscreen graphics. This eliminates the need for a surgical template, as traditionally used in image-guided surgery, and allows real-time correction during the drilling and insertion of the implant. While this technology is new and has little information about its accuracy, the potential is massive.

When to Use Image-Guided Surgery

When the patient and implant site are straightforward—such as an upper second premolar site in a low-smile-line patient with plenty of bone and attached gingiva—using an image-guided approach for a single implant does not offer a high return on investment. Image-guided surgery makes sense when there are challenges, such as anatomical limitations or multiple implants placed in the same jaw. Using a 3D-image-guided approach can save time in the operating room. However, it increases fees and possibly poses additional risks, as some studies have reported a lack of accuracy and higher complication rates. It is important to note that image-guided implant surgery has developed significantly in the last ten years, which explains the wide variation of outcomes in the literature. More outcome data on the various approaches to image-guided surgery is needed before its indications and contraindications are clear [1].

References

[1] Pozzi A, Polizzi G, Moy PK. Guided surgery with tooth-supported templates for single missing teeth: A critical review. *Eur J Oral Implantol*. 2016;9 Suppl 1:S135-53.

Chapter 20

Printed Surgical Template for Guided Implant Surgery

While manually fabricated templates (MFT) are produced in a dental laboratory using a system-specific drilling machine, stereolithographic templates (ST) are produced by computer-aided design and manufacturing technology. The latter is mainly performed in specialized milling centres. For most MFT and ST systems, it is mandatory to perform a three-dimensional radiography with a diagnostic (radiographic) template, including reference elements, which facilitate the transfer of the virtual sleeve positions into reality. The template fabrication for radiographic planning is costly and time-consuming. Recently, the coDiagnostiXTM software (Version 9.0, Dental Wings GmbH, Freiburg, Germany) was equipped with the option to design surgical templates for guided implant surgery without requiring a radiographic template and using three-dimensional printing technology for surgical template fabrication. A three-dimensional radiographic data set is uploaded into the planning software, which allows virtual implant planning. To transfer this planning into reality, a three-dimensional optical scan of a cast model (or intraoral scan) must be uploaded into the software and superimposed on radiographically visible matching references. Based on the optical scan, a virtual template framework can be included by mouse-click in the original planning. The sleeves can be included in the virtual framework, and the template is then printed with any home or office three-dimensional printer. However, though this technology improves template fabrication due to time and cost reductions, there is no data concerning the technical accuracy of this manufacturing approach.

Virtual Template Design

The cast models were equipped with three titanium pins, which were fixed to each cast model (Figure 41). These served as reference elements to evaluate the sleeve positioning and template printing accuracy, as described below.

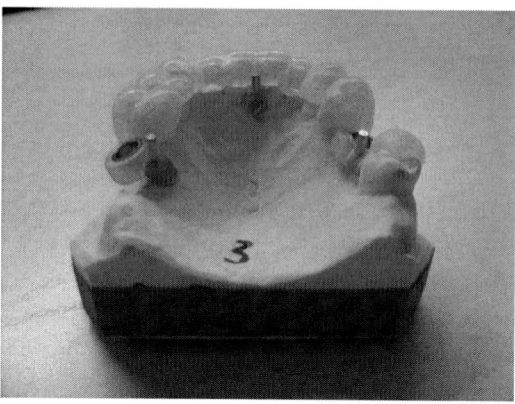

Figure 41. Printed template mounted on the original cast model equipped with three titanium pins for accuracy measurements.

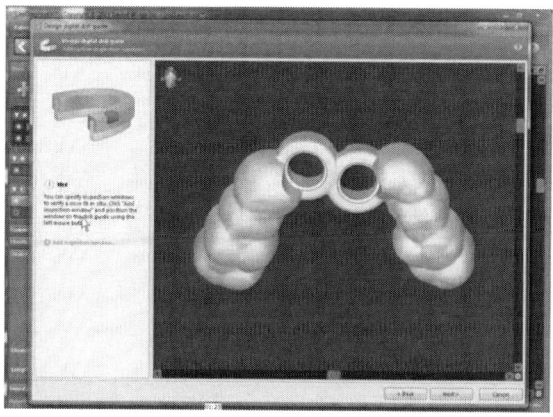

Figure 42. Virtually designed template with nots for the system-specific metal sleeves.

An optical scan of each cast model (including the titanium pins) was performed with a three-dimensional scanner (DW-3-90, Dental Wings Inc., Montreal, Canada). The data were transformed into Surface Tesselation Language (STL) files and uploaded into the coDiagnostiX software. The STL files of each patient were included in the original planning data by matching the scanned model with the three-dimensional radiography. This matching was based on anatomical landmarks, which were visible and mainly represented by natural teeth. Once the matching was completed, a virtual template, including the original sleeves for guidance, was designed using the three-dimensional scan of the model. Therefore, single points on each tooth's vestibular and oral sides, which indicate the direct contact zone of the virtual template on the teeth, were determined manually via mouse click. The software automatically connected these single points, creating the template's framework, including notations for the system-specific metal sleeves at the respective three-dimensional positions (Figure 42). Template Printing.

The designed virtual templates were exported as STL files and printed with a three-dimensional device (Objet Eden 260 V, Material: MED610, Stratasys Ltd., Minneapolis, MN, USA). For guided surgery, the system-specific metal sleeves with 5 mm diameter (T-sleeves, Institut Straumann AG, Basel, Switzerland) were manually pushed into the respective notches [1].

References

[1] Marjolein Vercruyssen TFGWR. Different techniques of static/dynamic guided implant surgery: Modalities and indications. *Periodontology*. 2014 October; 66.

Chapter 21

One Abutment One Time

Recent software advances offer the ability to combine CBCT and optically scanned data from high-quality diagnostic casts to perform CT-guided implant surgery and deliver a patient-specific CAD/CAM-milled abutment and non-occlusal function provisional at the same appointment, with ideal contours to maintain architecture. This abutment can remain in place and become the final abutment (where it is never removed, thus the "one-abutment, one-time" designation). Alternatively, it can be replaced with a new, digitally altered patient-specific abutment, thereby disrupting the implant-abutment interface only once because the dataset used to create the initial abutment can be referenced, modified, and redeveloped all within a digital environment without having to obtain a conventional impression.

Treatment Plan

After a collaborative workup between the surgical and restorative doctors, the patient decided to place an immediate implant and a prefabricated, patient specific abutment. A CBCT scan was obtained as part of the initial workup. The Digital Imaging Communication in Medicine (DICOMSM) data from this scan were then imported into the SIMPLANT® software (DENTSPLY Implants, www.dentsplyimplants.com) for virtual surgical planning. This plan incorporated an abutment core file, a virtual representation used to produce a custom ATLANTISTM abutment (DENTSPLY Implants) and the SIMPLANT Guide. Show the proposed implant site's initial clinical presentation and periapical radiograph, respectively. The clinical presentation was categorized as a case-type pattern (Pattern 1) implant candidate, revealing normal dental and surgical anatomy. Accordingly, to accurately represent the soft-tissue emergence profile inherent in the tissue around the existing tooth No. H, an irreversible hydrocolloid impression (Ivoclar Accu-Dent® System 2TM, Ivoclar Vivadent Inc., www.ivoclarvivadent.com) was made of the maxillary arch, and a diagnostic cast was created. The stone cast was optically scanned and registered to the CBCT hard tissue data in the SIMPLANT planning software and its accompanying CAD/CAM workflow process. Figure 43 shows the virtual representation of this optical scan, with a virtual replacement tooth generated from the SIMPLANT software. A known angle correction was virtually incorporated into the planned implant path. Figure 44 shows the cross-sectional view of the axial inclination and the required existing axis of the planned final tooth position.

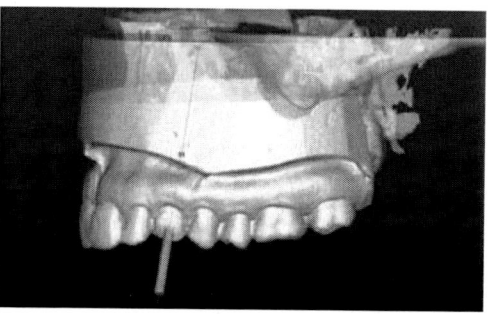

Figure 43. Digital image of optically scanned maxillary diagnostic cast, with virtually designed replacement tooth and proposed axis.

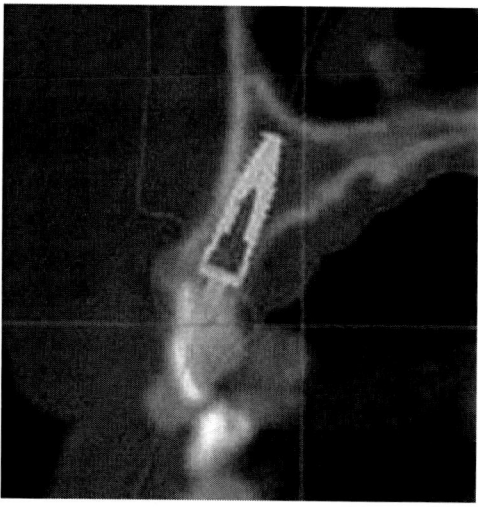

Figure 44. Conebeam computed tomographic cross-section showing degree of correction required from existing axis of tooth No. H. Optimal thickness of bone at the alveolar crest is evident.

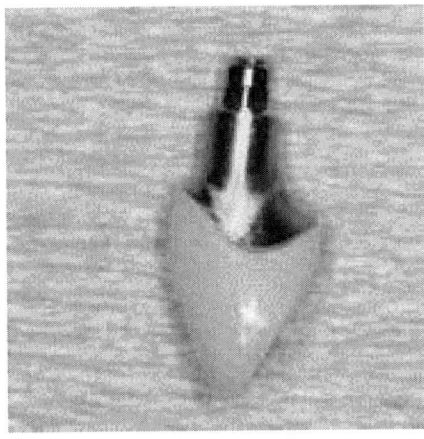

Figure 45. CAD/CAM-milled PMMA provisional seated on abutment.

A Patient-specific abutment that was virtually created the milled patient-specific gold-shaded titanium abutment and polymethylmethacrylate (PMMA) provisional created by the laboratory through the digital workflow process (using the virtual design data) are shown separately and seated (Figure 45).

Surgical Procedure

Under intravenous conscious sedation and local anaesthesia, a sulcular incision was made with a microsurgical straight blade to remove the supra-crestal fibres, followed by an uneventful atraumatic extraction of tooth No. H. After extraction, the complete seating of the surgical guide (Tapered Navigator® SIMPLANT SAFE Guide®, DENTSPLY Implants) was verified. The osteotomy site was then completed through the Tapered Navigator SIMPLANT SAFE Guide CT-guided System using a flapless approach. A 4/3 Biomet *3i* T3 Tapered Prevail® implant (Biomet *3i*, www.biomet3i.com) was delivered through the Tapered Navigator SIMPLANT SAFE Guide using the appropriate implant mount for totally guided implant surgery. The Tapered Navigator, SIMPLANT SAFE Guide system, has rotational timing, which allows for the implant hex orientation to be positioned at the time of surgery as it was oriented during the pre-surgical fabrication of the abutment. The vertical positioning was confirmed and verified with a UNC-15 mm periodontal probe. An objective analysis was used to substantiate initial implant stability. It shows an Osstell® ISQ Smartpeg (Osstell AB, www.osstell.com), which uses resonance frequency to assess implant stability, represented by the implant stability quotient (ISQ). The implant trajectory is also clearly observed by the engagement of the SmartPeg with the implant. This implant's observed ISQ value of 80 indicates high stability (Figure 46). A facial view of the seated patient-specific ATLANTIS abutment, with its appropriately positioned screw-access hole.

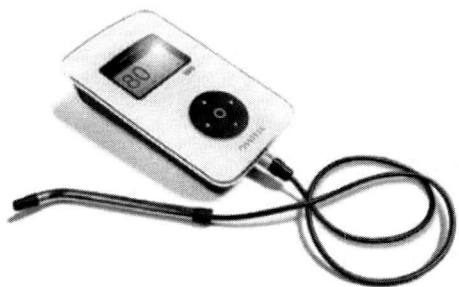

Figure 46. Smartpeg.

Postoperative Treatment

Good initial and mid-phase soft-tissue healing was evident one week postoperatively, with excellent preservation of the gingival margin. At five weeks, limited gingival inflammation was present due to the patient's lack of optimal plaque control. At 14 weeks, the peri-implant soft tissue health was improved, and osseointegration was confirmed clinically and radiographically. The soft-tissue architecture was well maintained for 14 weeks postoperatively. With the provisional non-occlusal function removed, good peri-implant soft-tissue tone was evident from facial and palatal aspects. Notably, the incisal view showed healthy sulcular epithelium, indicating good biologic-width maturation, confirmed radiographically in the osseous topography. The 14-week radiographic view of the implant and abutment shows good maintenance of crestal bone with an established biologic-width formation, suggesting complete osseointegration. Slight exposure of the abutment-provisional margin that had occurred on the mesial aspect A final abutment was designed between the restorative office and the laboratory using a digital workflow to adjust the margin virtually with no disruption of the implant-abutment junction or the newly established biologic width. The initial (green) and revised (blue) virtual abutments and associated margin designs. The final ATLANTIS abutment and crown (IPS e.max® CeramIvoclar Vivadent; ArgenZTM milled zirconia, Argen Corp.) were delivered afterwards [1].

References

[1] Van de Wiele G, Teughels W, Vercruyssen M, Coucke W, Temmerman A, Quirynen M. The accuracy of guided surgery via mucosa-supported stereolithographic surgical templates in the hands of surgeons with little experience. *Clinical oral implants research*. 2015 Dec;26(12):1489-94.

Chapter 22

Teeth in an Hour

In this application, the full potential of the dual function of the surgical template is used to pre-produce the restorative solution before implant surgery. This provides an absolute, immediate functional treatment result. The reconstituted master cast is used to construct the planned prosthetic option, either retrievable screw-retained guided abutment bridge construction or a cemented bridge on customized zirconia Procera abutments. Either solution may be definitive or provisional. Definitive screw-retained prostheses utilize a Procera titanium implant bridge framework veneered with either plastic crown and bridge material or titanium-compatible ceramic material. Provisional screw-retained prostheses are constructed with acrylic resin, incorporating appropriate sleeves to anchor guided abutments. As a provisional procedure, cemented solutions can utilize definitive Procera zirconia frameworks veneered with NobelRondo zirconia porcelain or acrylic bridgework. The determination of paths, whether definitive or provisional, depends upon evaluating multiple factors. Final pathway Teeth-in-an-hour restorations offer minimal flexibility and higher risk in aesthetically demanding situations. Provisional pathway restorations offer the advantage of giving the clinician and patient time to evaluate aesthetic and functional results, particularly in situations of high aesthetic demand, thus facilitating the opportunity to satisfy patient expectations. Thus, flexibility is maximized, stress is reduced, and the necessity to remake final restorations is minimized. These advantages are further enhanced in situations requiring secondary soft tissue manipulation in high-end aesthetic cases [1].

References

[1] Zitzmann NU, Margolin MD, Filippi A, Weiger R, Krastl G. Patient assessment and diagnosis in implant treatment. *Australian Dental Journal*. 2008 Jun;53:S3-10.

Chapter 23

Clinical Outcome of Guided Implant Surgery

Implant Survival

Since 2010, several reviews, including systematic reviews, have assessed the accuracy of flapless-guided surgery in clinical studies. The implant survival rate generally ranges from 91% to 100%. In a review by Tahmaseb et al. as part of the 2013 International Team for Implantology consensus conference, 14 survival and 24 accuracy studies were included. The overall implant survival rate was reported to be 97.3% based on 1941 implants. However, in 36.4% of cases, intra-operative or prosthetic complications were reported. Those included template fractures during surgery, a change of plan because of limited implant stability, the need for nonplanned grafting, prosthetic screw loosening, misfits, and prosthesis fractures. Based on the meta-analysis, the authors concluded that there is, as yet, no evidence suggesting that computer-assisted surgery is superior to conventional surgery in terms of safety, outcome, morbidity, or efficiency. D'haese et al. reviewed 31 clinical studies, of which 10 reported accuracy. They concluded that guided surgery yields a more accurate placement than freehand implant placement.

Nevertheless, from both cadaver and clinical studies, it was obvious that guided surgery needs to be more accurate. Deviations at the shoulder of the implant hamper the correct fit of the suprastructures and could require extensive adaptations in occlusion and articulation. They suggest that a 2-mm safety zone should be respected apically to the planned position to avoid critical anatomic structures. There are a few reviews assessing implant survival with flapless and guided surgery. Voulgarakis et al. evaluated the outcome of three treatment protocols: freehand surgery, guided surgery with a prosthetic stent, and guided surgery with stereolithographic computer-guided navigation. They included 23 studies with a prospective or retrospective design, but randomized control trials were unavailable, and the significant heterogeneity of the studies excluded a meta-analysis. Lin et al. (35) focused on the clinical results of flapless surgery. They performed a meta-analysis on implant survival and peri-implant bone loss based on 12 studies, including seven randomized controlled clinical trials. The meta-analysis of

Moraschini et al. (40) reported on survival, crestal bone, and complications with guided surgery based on 13 studies. The implant survival, as reported in the three reviews, ranges from 89% to 100%, albeit the follow-up time is relatively short, ranging from 6 to 48 months. Based on a total of 35 clinical trials, it can be concluded that freehand surgery is comparable to guided flapless surgery in terms of implant survival, marginal bone remodelling, and peri-implant variables.

Accuracy

Computer-guided implant procedures have often been recommended in critical anatomic situations (e.g., an implant to be placed adjacent to the mandibular nerve). Therefore, knowledge of the potential maximal implant deviation of these systems is highly relevant to daily clinical practice and must be considered. The data analyzed in the proceedings of the 5th International Team for Implantology Consensus Conference on computer-guided surgery showed an inaccuracy at the implant entry point (between the planned implant position and the position at which the implant was inserted) of, on average, 1.12 mm (maximum 4.5 mm) and an inaccuracy of, on average, 1.39 mm at the apex of implants (maximum 4.5 mm).7.1 mm). However, the maximal deviations measured in the two studies were far outside the acceptable range. These outliers might be related to external factors. For example, Di Giacomo et al. proposed that movements of the surgical guide might cause differences in the deviation during implant preparation. This group suggested further improvements that could provide better template stability during surgery for unilateral bone-supported and non-tooth-supported templates. Moreover, sandblasted with large grit acid-etched (computer-assisted manufacture) guides had slightly better accuracy than laboratory guides (noncomputer-assisted manufacture). However, the number of cases was significantly lower for the noncomputer-assisted manufacturing group (171 implants vs. 1,569 implants). Furthermore, the supporting structures have a significant impact on accuracy. Tahmaseb et al. showed that guides supported by mini-implants provided high accuracy in implant positioning. This might result from the reproducibility of the template position during the acquisition of radiographic data and implantation. This is especially true in fully edentulous patients for whom no other references are available. Moreover, clinical studies have shown a statistically significant lower accuracy for bone-supported guides than other support modes. These results could also explain why the flapped approaches had lower accuracy than the flapless ones, as most treatments in which a flap is raised use bone-supported surgical guides [1].

Complications

Various early surgical and prosthetic complications have been reported in the literature when computer-guided surgery is applied. The most frequently reported complications are related to intra-operatively broken stereolithographic surgical guides, alterations to the surgical plan, early implant loss because of a lack of primary stability, and prosthetic fracture. Schneider et al. reported an incidence of 9.1% for early surgical complications and an incidence of 18.8% for early prosthetic complications. These complications are associated with incorrect implant placement or deviations from the originally planned location. This occurs especially when stereolithographic-guided surgery is followed by immediate provisionalization with a previously prepared fixed bridge. Additionally, late prosthetic complications were found in 12% of patients. A metaanalysis revealed that the mean horizontal deviations were 1.1–1.6 mm, but with higher maximal deviations. In particular, the higher deviations may cause nerve disturbances, damage anatomically vital structures (such as the sinuses and nose), and additionally lead to prosthetic complications [2].

References

[1] Solow RA. Simplified radiographic-surgical template for placement of multiple, parallel implants. *The Journal of prosthetic dentistry*. 2001 Jan 1;85(1):26-9..

[2] Hultin M, Svensson KG, Trulsson M. Clinical advantages of computer-guided implant placement: a systematic review. *Clinical oral implants research*. 2012 Oct;23:124-35.

Chapter 24

Artificial Intelligence and Guided Implant Surgery

A plethora of advancements in technology during the last few decades have integrated these technological advancements into our day-to-day lives. Artificial intelligence (AI) is a field of engineering science dealing with computers' computational understanding and ability to mimic the human brain to exhibit intelligent behavior and perform tasks effortlessly. Artificial intelligence (AI) can be loosely defined as the study of algorithms that give machines the ability to reason and perform cognitive functions such as problem-solving, object and word recognition, and decision-making. It has begun to establish itself even in dentistry and medicine. The introduction of virtual reality in medicine and dentistry, from data acquisition to even performing virtual surgeries, was made possible. The need for proper documentation of the patient's information and quick and reliable treatment protocols through robotics in the field of surgery has encouraged using these software technologies to assist the dentist in diagnosing and treating patients efficiently.

The elegance of AI is that machines can be trained to evaluate large data sets and memorize them to impart the most favorable diagnoses. Artificial intelligence-based virtual dental companions can perform different tasks in routine dental practice with fewer human resources, fewer errors, and greater precision than humans. It guides in coordinating appointments, executing insurance and paperwork, and assisting in clinical diagnosis or treatment planning. It also helps inform the dental practitioner about the subject's medical history and habits, like smoking and alcoholism. Especially in dental emergencies, when the practitioner is unavailable, the patient has the option of emergency teleassistance, which would benefit the patient.

AI has become a part of our daily lives. With the advent of Siri and Alexa, we are now used to voice commands. The dental practice has also been updated from the use of touch-sensitive dental chairs to voice-controlled dental chairs that do not need any manual input from the clinicians. The chair positions, water dispensing, and light control can be efficiently handled based on the voice command. Furthermore, a relatively sterile clinical examination form can be practiced with a reduced risk of cross-contamination during treatments. Thus, a detailed virtual database of the patient can be created, which will go a long way in providing ideal treatment for the patient.

AI software programs have assisted the surgeon in planning surgeries with reduced operation time, thereby preserving the vital structures to the smallest detail before the surgery with higher intraoperative accuracy. One more fruitful clinical application is image-guided surgeries that allow for further accurate surgical resection, possibly decreasing the need for revision procedures. In AI, "intelligent agents" observe and learn from their environment. Based on their learning, they then perform actions to achieve their goals with the maximum chance of success. AI is primarily expected in scenarios where automated cognitive learning and problem-solving are expected. Due to the complex nature of human tissue interaction and a lack of awareness about the possible competencies of computational tactics in surgical practice, AI has taken longer to enter the clinical surgery domain. However, AI is now rapidly advancing. The potential effect expected from artificial intelligence in medical surgery is to foil rather than substitute for human skills. Complex decision-making processes that could include, for instance, the choices about organ-preserving vs. radical surgery, the timing of surgery, and the need for multimodal therapy are involved in a surgical process. Furthermore, the surgeons should provide personalized patient data on the likelihood of mortality or morbidity and other potential risks. An elegant solution for such cases could be provided by the growth of tools such as algorithmic medical decision support within surgery, fortified by multiparametric data amalgamation and allowing communication between the computer systems and data stores.

In guided surgery during head and neck imaging modalities, AI provides an added advantage due to its distinctive learning ability. It can be assimilated with other imaging modalities like CBCT and MRI to determine infinitesimal deviations from normality that could have gone unrecognized by the human eye. Illustrations include the definite location of landmarks on radiographs, which aids in the location of minor apical foramen, the detection of vertical root fractures, and cephalometric analysis, thereby strengthening the accuracy of working length determination. The Logicon Caries Detector helps in the detection and characterization of proximal caries. Economically, all these could be translated into better patient care.

The field of artificial intelligence has transformed medicine and dentistry in several ways. Though artificial intelligence systems are a great asset in dentistry and dental education, the human biological system is complex, and it is to be noted that these technological advancements are still the brainchild of innovations and discoveries by humankind. Furthermore, AI can only assist the clinician in performing the tasks efficiently but in no way replace the intellect of human knowledge, skill, and treatment planning. AI is expanding its footprint in clinical systems ranging from databases to intraoperative video analysis. The unique nature of surgical practice leaves surgeons well-positioned to help usher in the next phase of AI, one focused on generating evidence-based, real-time clinical decision support designed to optimize patient care and surgeon workflow.

Chapter 25

Conclusion

Surgical models and guidance have acquired a new dimension by integrating CAD/CAM technology and computer-guided surgery. With the advent of low-radiation cone-beam computed tomography, now available in small practical units, access to CT data is simplified, and, in turn, advanced diagnosis and the fabrication of CAD/CAM surgical guides become more realistic. Precision has been improved, and uncertainty and surgical time have been reduced, thus addressing complex rehabilitation more confidently. In addition, predictable positioning allows for a better prosthetic outcome by simplifying abutment selection and avoiding complex laboratory fabrication when misalignment must be corrected. In addition, novel techniques are emerging that enable the preparation of the final prosthesis before implant placement. Precise guidance is crucial to such complex reconstruction, so minimal adaptation is performed after surgery. Future technical improvements will allow dentists to access these technologies while controlling costs, reducing surgical time, and minimizing restorative steps.

New technologies based on the 3D evaluation of patients for dental implants have opened new avenues to clinicians for accurate and predictable diagnosis, planning, and treatment in a multidisciplinary patient-based approach. Communication between clinicians and understanding these technologies are vital to improving case results and clinical outcomes. Analyzing, understanding, and adopting these technologies will open new doors for the dental team and benefit patients with more predictable outcomes. CT-guided implant planning and placement do not remove the need for the surgical and restorative teams to diligently adhere to the basic principles of implant surgery and prosthetic dentistry. It is imperative to uphold and adhere to established principles in various aspects of implant dentistry, such as implant spacing, depth, and angulation, case planning and engineering, minimally traumatic manipulation of soft and hard tissues, soft tissue and bone grafting, healing time for osseointegration, soft and hard tissue healing, heat generation, dental materials, ideal occlusion, and numerous other factors. CT-guided implant surgery facilitates the placement of dental implants in an ideal position according to a restoratively driven treatment plan. The final tooth position is determined first. The ideal implant position is then planned, and the implant is placed in that position precisely. Treatment plans should be created according to the requirements of an individual case and the comfort level of the surgical and restorative teams. Cases can be treated with implants staged with healing abutments or immediately loaded with temporary, or in some circumstances, final, restorations.

Proper case selection and patient awareness, education, and compliance are all critical factors for success. A steep learning curve often exists before successfully incorporating CT-guided surgery into a dental implant practice. Clinicians interested in these technologies are strongly encouraged to pursue continuing education. CT-guided implant surgery is not conventional implant surgery. Knowledge of CT scans, proprietary treatment planning software, complete treatment protocols, and guided surgery instrumentation and surgical techniques are all instrumental to a successful outcome. In addition, clinicians should consider the inherent costs involved in using proprietary software and CAD/CAM processing technologies. Good patient selection and appropriate diagnosis, planning, and treatment are of primary importance. These requirements are best facilitated by knowledge of CT-based technologies enabling the clinician to adhere to surgical, prosthetic, and biological principles that optimize patient care.

About the Authors

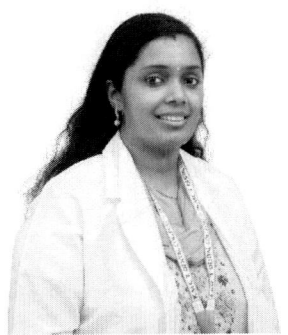

Niveditha S. Prasad
KMCT Dental College,
KUHS University, Kerala, India

Dr Niveditha S. Prasad received her BDS degree from MES Dental College, Calicut University in 2016 and MDS from KMCT Dental College, KUHS University in 2020. Now, she is working as assistant professor at KMCT Dental College, KUHS University. She has received First prize in poster presentation in National IPS convention, First prize in paper presentation in Midterm State conference – Post graduate convention. She has achieved Dr Jacob Hyson award for best scientific Article – Indian Prosthodontic Society Kerala state branch. She is a Principal investigator in ongoing research projects at SERB (Science and Engineering Research Board) Govt. of India and Co- Investigator in research grant at KSCSTE, Govt of Kerala. She actively participated/attended many IPS National & state Conferences and Conventions. She has conducted a Pre-conference course based on CBCT evaluation of implantology at Conference held at Hyderabad. She has various publications in National and International Journals.

Email: nivedithaprasad8@gmail.com.

About the Authors

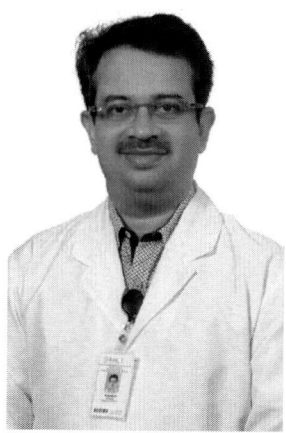

M. Sheejith
KMCT Dental College,
KUHS University, Kerala, India

Dr. M Sheejith completed his BDS from Yenepoya Dental College, Mangalore, Karnataka (affiliated to Rajiv Gandhi University of Health Sciences) in 1999, and MDS in Prosthodontics from the prestigious Government Dental College, Calicut, Kerala (affiliated to Calicut University) in 2006. He also completed PGCOI from College of Dental Surgery, Manipal, Karnataka in 2013, and PGCE from Meenakshi Ammal Dental College, Chennai, Tamil Nadu in 2012. A keen Academician, an astute Clinician, and an exemplary Speaker, he has been at the forefront of Prosthodontic and Implant Dentistry as a Mentor & Educator with numerous International & National Publications to his credit. Currently, he is working as Professor and Head in the Department of Prosthodontics at KMCT Dental College, Calicut with more than 15 years of Teaching Experience. He serves as a PG Guide under Kerala University of Health Sciences, and an Internal as well as External Examiner to various Universities in the country. He is an Editorial Board Member of IPS Kerala Journal and was an Executive Committee Member of IPS Kerala State branch. He is also a Life-time Member of Indian Prosthodontics Society (IPS), Indian Society of Prosthodontics-Restorative-Periodontics (ISPRP), and Indian Dental Association (IDA).

Email: sheejithm2000@yahoo.co.in.

About the Authors

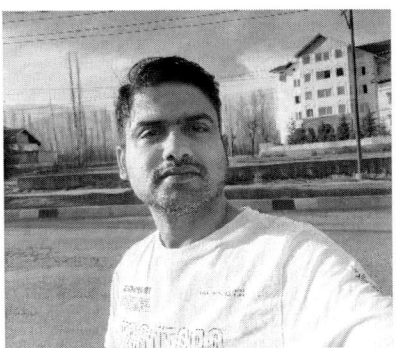

Raj V. S. Sarath
IQRAA International Hospital,
Calicut, Kerala, India

Raj V. S. Sarath is a consultant Radiologist of IQRAA International Hospital and research centre. He has done his MBBS from government medical college, Trivandrum, Kerala, India, DMRD from Pusphagiri Institute of Medical Science and DNB from KMCT dental college, Calicut, Kerala, India. He actively participated/attended many National & state Conferences and Conventions. He has various publications in National and International Journals. He actively takes part in research activities held at the hospital.
Email: sarathrajvs@gmail.com

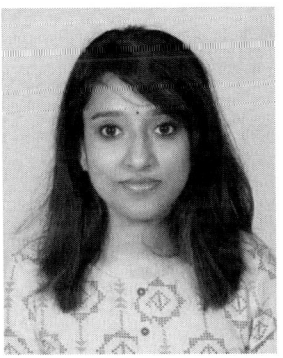

Nivea T. Francis
KMCT Dental College,
KUHS University, Kerala, India

Dr. Nivea T. Francis received her bachelor's degree from Rajarajeswari Dental College and Hospital, Rajiv Gandhi University of Health Sciences, in

2012 and her master's degree from Rajiv Gandhi University of Health Sciences in 2016. Now, she is working as assistant professor at KMCT Dental College, KUHS University.

Email: nivfra90@gmail.com.

Index

A

abutment, v, 8, 24, 31, 33, 36, 38, 40, 41, 56, 73, 74, 85, 86, 99, 101, 102, 105, 115
accuracy, v, 3, 4, 7, 8, 11, 12, 13, 14, 15, 16, 19, 22, 23, 32, 51, 53, 70, 82, 86, 88, 90, 91, 93, 95, 96, 103, 107, 108, 112
Advanced template, 55, 56
advantages, 7, 11, 15, 23, 53, 59, 63, 83, 105, 109
allografts, 1
anatomage guide, 43, 44
Artificial intelligence (AI), v, 111, 112, 113
ATLANTIS™ abutment, 99

B

Basic template, 55, 56
block grafts, 1
bone morphogenic proteins (BMP 2), 1
bone volume, 21, 80, 83
bone-supported, 62, 84, 108

C

cast based guided implant surgery, 77
CBCT guided flapless implant surgery (CBCT guided), 83
completely limiting design, 57
complications, v, 3, 29, 90, 92, 107, 108, 109
Compu-Guide Template System, 55
computed tomography (CT), 1, 3, 7, 8, 11, 12, 13, 14, 15, 19, 20, 21, 27, 29, 50, 51, 52, 55, 56, 59, 60, 61, 68, 69, 70, 72, 77, 99, 101, 115, 116
Compu-Temp template, 55, 56

computer-aided manufacturing (CAD/CAM), 1, 3, 4, 11, 12, 13, 15, 54, 58, 72, 87, 99, 100, 101, 115, 116
cone beam computed tomography (CBCT), v, 4, 5, 7, 19, 21, 61, 69, 83, 84, 86, 87, 90, 99, 112, 117
cone beam radiographic scanning technology, 1
cone beam volumetric tomography (CBVT), 7
CT based guided implant surgery, 69

D

data acquisition, 69, 111
DENTSPLY implants, 13, 99, 101
diagnosis, 2, 4, 8, 23, 35, 48, 63, 105, 111, 115, 116
Digital Imaging Communication in Medicine (DICOM™), 99
disadvantages, 7, 15, 27, 53, 59
distraction osteogenesis, 1

F

fixed prosthesis type 1 (FP-1), 40, 42
fixed prosthesis type 2 (FP-2), 40
fixed prosthesis type 3 (FP-3), 41
flapless and open flap procedures, 17
free-handed surgery, 84
fully-guided surgery, 85

G

guided bone regeneration techniques (GBR), 1
guided implant surgery, v, vii, 3, 4, 11, 14, 15, 16, 17, 19, 20, 22, 23, 27, 29, 33, 53,

61, 62, 63, 68, 71, 82, 90, 93, 95, 97, 99, 101, 107, 115, 116
guided surgery, v, 1, 3, 4, 11, 15, 19, 23, 24, 29, 31, 46, 54, 61, 62, 64, 67, 69, 83, 85, 86, 89, 90, 93, 97, 103, 107, 108, 109, 112, 115, 116
guided surgical templates, 35, 36

I

identification, 69
image guided implant surgery, v, 87
implant placement, 2, 3, 4, 5, 8, 11, 12, 13, 14, 15, 17, 19, 20, 21, 22, 24, 30, 31, 32, 33, 36, 37, 40, 42, 43, 46, 48, 56, 57, 68, 77, 82, 83, 86, 89, 91, 93, 107, 109, 115
implant position, 2, 3, 9, 11, 12, 19, 20, 21, 22, 40, 42, 56, 63, 64, 65, 72, 74, 84, 87, 108, 116
implant prosthodontics, 1, 8, 9
implant survival, v, 12, 83, 107
inferior alveolar nerve (IAN), 4, 20, 24

L

Laney-Poitras template, 39

M

manually fabricated templates (MFT), 95
manufacturer-specific master sleeves, 45, 47
Med 3-D, 23, 29, 30, 31, 33
Med 3-D AG, 29
minimal bone, 24
mucosa-supported, 62

N

narrow ridges, 17, 24
navigation, 4, 5, 64, 68, 69, 70, 83, 93, 107
NobelGuide protocols, 13
NobelGuide surgical templates, 12, 13
NobelGuide system (Nobel Biocare), 12, 15, 24, 29, 30, 72, 73, 74

non-resorbable, 1

P

Pilot Surgiguide, 46
platelet-enriched plasma (PRP), 1
postoperative treatment, v, 102
prosthetic planning, 35
protocols, 1, 31, 60, 61, 63, 107, 111, 116

R

registration, 11, 15, 33, 61, 69, 70
resorbable, 1, 85
robotic surgery, v, 93

S

SAFE SurgiGuide, 47
SAFE SurgiTemplates, 47
SimPlant, 8, 9, 10, 13, 23, 29, 30, 31, 32, 33, 43, 47, 60, 62, 63
SIMPLANT® software, 99
sinus grafts, 1
stereolithographic templates (ST), 50, 74, 77, 95
surgical accuracy, v, 90
surgical guides, 11, 12, 13, 14, 42, 43, 44, 48, 49, 50, 58, 60, 62, 83, 87, 88, 92, 109, 115
surgical phases, 35
surgical template, v, 9, 11, 12, 13, 14, 15, 23, 24, 27, 30, 33, 35, 36, 37, 38, 43, 48, 49, 50, 52, 53, 55, 56, 57, 58, 62, 63, 65, 66, 67, 71, 72, 74, 93, 95, 103, 105, 109

U

universal master sleeves, 44
Universal Surgiguide, 46
universal templates, 46

V

virtual implant planning, 11, 63, 95
virtual template design, v, 95

X

xenografts, 1